THE BEGINNER'S GUIDE TO
ESSENTIAL OILS
ANCIENT MEDICINE

Dr. Josh Axe
Jordan Rubin
Ty Bollinger

ISBN-13: 978-0-7684-5191-7

ISBN-13 eBook: 978-0-7684-5192-4

Printed in the USA

     5 6 / 24 23 22

CONTENTS

INTRODUCTION

HEALING WITH BIBLICAL MEDICINE

Let's travel back in time to over 3,000 years ago to visit the palace of King David in Israel's capital city, Jerusalem. You explore the immense castle until you stumble upon the private chambers of the king and discover a large cupboard. You've found King David's medicine cabinet! You swing open the heavy wooden doors, locate a treasure trove of healing balms, oils, spices and herbs inside, and you decide to take a closer look.

First, you find the woodsy and sweet-smelling sandalwood, which the king may use to clean wounds or as a natural aphrodisiac. Then you find some minty tasting hyssop that King David likely uses to soothe his aching muscles after battle and which acts as a powerful antiseptic. You smell the distinctive aroma of clean, energizing cypress, known for its ability to heal wounds and infections and serve as a powerful deodorant to keep the king smelling fresh in between his royal baths. You find smoky, bittersweet, sticky myrrh that the king and his royal family use to fight aging and help prevent gum disease. Then you pick up a vial of warm, spicy cassia, which boosts the body's immune system as it acts as a natural insect repellant to keep the king from being harassed by bugs during the hot Jerusalem summers. And finally, you find highly cherished and prized frankincense that King David uses in his and his wives' soaps and perfumes to hydrate and protect their bodies.

All of these oils and more are what the queens and kings of ancient days used as their medicine. There were no pharmacies on every corner; instead, there were simply herbs, spices and other plant parts known to promote health and healing.

Fast forward to today and step into our own personal homes. Inside, we invite you to look into our medicine cabinets. What you won't find is a single prescription medication. Instead, you will discover a cornucopia of ancient medicines and natural remedies based in nature, including herbs, spices, supplements and dozens of essential oils. Inside Dr. Josh's home, you'll always find frankincense; Jordan is never far away from a bottle of lavender; and Ty's office is drenched in the aromas of orange and peppermint.

We use essential oils in extensive ways in our lives; they wear many hats, if you will—as our medicines, our cleansing agents, our personal care products and countless other uses. Why do we rely on essential oils exactly, and why do we believe that everyone else should, too?

The reasons are simple: Instead of simply depending on prescription medications and synthetic drugs with a list of dangerous side effects, our families have opted for safer, natural remedies with thousands of years of history proving their benefits. Instead of using common household cleaners and personal care products that contain ingredients that cause toxicity, we have chosen superior alternatives that can achieve the same (or even better) results without the risk of damaging our bodies.

In the quest for health and vibrant living, the three of us have collaborated multiple times over the last several years in order to share important messages of health and hope. During this time, we have discovered that we all believe essential oils are one of the most powerful forms of plant-based medicine in the world. Now, we want to show you how essential oils can transform the health of your entire family.

Essential oils can serve innumerable functions in your life—from fostering relaxation and caring for scrapes to helping fight disease and promoting healing.

Essential oils were placed on this Earth to benefit our health and provide rejuvenation. In fact, they have been a vital part of our individual journeys, both personally and in the pursuit of helping others find abundant health.

Allow us to share the roles essential oils play in our personal lives in order to equip and empower you to use them every day.

We have seen essential oils benefit our families and our patients in some of the following ways:

- **Reduce toxicity**
- **Balance hormones**
- **Improve digestion**
- **Boost energy**
- **Improve brain function**
- **Reduce emotional stress**
- **Produce radiant skin**
- **Boost immunity and fight infections**
- **Alleviate aches and pains**

And, a whole lot more!

USING ESSENTIAL OILS SAFELY AND EFFECTIVELY

Everyone has a different "essential oil style." Some people use essential oils as natural remedies while others use them to fragrance the air. Some use them to replace toxic personal care products. Finally, other people use essential oils for everything—it becomes part of their cleaning products, shampoo, toothpaste, detergent, deodorant and used as first aid remedies.

The three of us have our own essential own styles that are unique to our families.

Jordan has seen his life transformed by the use of essential oils every day. His essential oil style might be called "ancient healing." As he anoints his family with oils each morning, he is reminded of the wondrous power within the oils as he thanks the Great Physician who created them.

Ty's essential oil style is one of "soothing air." He prefers to diffuse his oils because he believes that is the best way for his entire family to experience the immune boosting, restorative, energizing abilities of essential oils each and every day.

Dr. Josh enjoys finding new ways to use essential oils. His essential oil style is "infinite possibilities" because he and his wife use it to clean their air, care for their dogs, improve their sleep, stop headaches, improve concentration and countless other uses.

What's your essential oil style? Everybody has one—even those who are just beginning to explore the world of essential oils. The good news is that there are so many oils and so many ways to use them that the options for use are virtually limitless.

There are, however, a finite number of ways essential oils may be used when it comes to our bodies. The ways in which they are used are dependent upon the needs or desired outcome of the individual using the oil. This chapter will describe the three main methods of essential oil use: 1) aromatherapy applications (direct inhalation and diffusing), 2) topical use and 3) internal use.

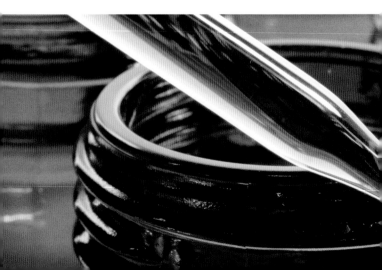

THE FRAGRANT WORLD OF AROMATHERAPY

The aromatic nature of essential oils stimulates powerful mental, emotional and physiologic responses. Not only does the aroma of the natural essential oil stimulate the brain to trigger a reaction, but also when inhaled into the lungs, the naturally occurring chemicals can supply therapeutic benefits. For example, diffusing eucalyptus essential oil is an effective way to help ease congestion.

When a person simply breathes in the aroma of an essential oil, this is called direct inhalation. Here are some methods of **direct inhalation:**

» Open an essential oil bottle and breathe in the aroma.

» Place a drop or two of oil or a blend of oils in the hands, rub them together, make a cup around the nose and mouth and breathe in. (Note: Use caution when practicing this method. Some essential oils require prior mixing with

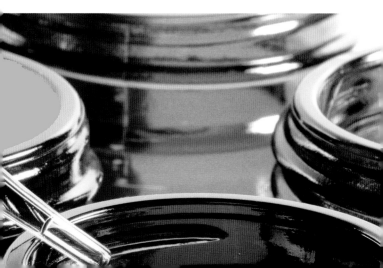

a carrier oil, such as coconut oil, to dilute the concentration and prevent skin irritation.)

» Place a drop or two of oil or a blend of oils on a piece of cloth or tissue, hold it close to the face and inhale.

Another popular method of aromatherapy is **diffusing essential oils** into a room. When using a diffuser, the essential oil is evaporated into the surrounding environment. Diffusing essential oils can alter your mood by relaxing or stimulating the mind. It can also kill airborne pathogens and treat a respiratory condition. Here are some ways to diffuse essential oils:

» To clean the air, add a blend of lemon, clove, orange, cinnamon, eucalyptus and rosemary oils to a diffuser.

» To improve energy, add peppermint to a diffuser.

» To reduce stress or combat a headache, or just to relax, add lavender to a diffuser.

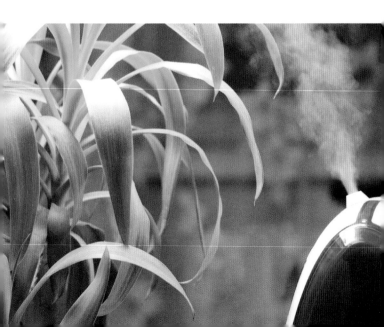

THERE ARE FOUR MAIN TYPES OF DIFFUSERS:

1 **Atomizing:** No water is involved when using atomizing diffusers—the essential oil bottle is connected to the diffuser to create a pure vapor that is extremely powerful and therapeutic.

2 **Vaporizing:** These diffusers use water with the essential oil; ultrasonic waves are used to emit the oil and water particles into the air. Vaporizing diffusers are very quiet, so they are popular with therapists, yoga instructors and other professionals who are looking to achieve a peaceful environment.

3 **Fan or evaporative:** Evaporative diffusers are usually lower in cost and used in a smaller area. A fan blows air from the room through a pad or filter that has essential oils on it. The air blowing through the pad causes the oils to evaporate more quickly than with other diffusers, and the air with the evaporated oil is blown into the room.

4 **Heat:** Like evaporative diffusers, heat diffusers also cause the essential oils to evaporate quickly; these diffusers use heat instead of blowing air to accomplish diffusion.

Another way to diffuse a room with essential oils is by using a **spray bottle.** Oils can be mixed with water or alcohol and then sprayed in the air, on surfaces or on the body. This will create a refreshing and energizing environment.

LET'S GET TOPICAL

When essential oils are **applied directly to the skin,** they are absorbed and enter the bloodstream (this is because the oils are fat-soluble). When an oil is applied to the skin with no carrier oil, this is called a "neat" application. The soles of the feet is one area of the body that is sometimes exposed to a neat application. It is also one of the most popular places to apply oils. There are several reasons for this:

Less irritation. When oils are administered on the soles of the feet, there is a lower risk of skin irritation. The skin there is less sensitive than the skin on the rest of the body.

No sebum. The soles of the feet and the palms of the hands are the only sites on our body without sebaceous glands. Sebum is an oily substance that helps lubricate and waterproof the skin. Since the palms and the soles do not secrete sebum, they are more ready to absorb oil.

Bypass the liver. When you apply oils to the soles of the feet, the oils bypass the liver and will not accumulate there. Instead of being processed by the liver, the oils reach the lower bronchial capillaries via the circulatory system and the entire organism unprocessed.

Other key points of application on the body include behind the ears, neck, abdomen, upper back, temples and along the spine. When applying essential oils, sensitive skin areas should be avoided, such as the eyes, inner ears, genitals and open skin.

Essential oils are commonly **combined with a carrier oil,** which not only dilutes the essential oil but also prevents easy evaporation. Because using a carrier oil dilutes the potency of the essential oil being used, the chances of experiencing an irritation or skin reaction are reduced. Some of the best carrier oils include coconut oil, jojoba oil, grapeseed oil, olive oil, almond oil, pomegranate seed oil and avocado oil:

▶ **Coconut oil**—The best all-purpose oil to use in personal care products, from making homemade body care products like lotion, deodorant and toothpaste to diluting for topical use. When used topically, fractionated coconut oil works best due to its liquid state at room temperature.

▶ **Jojoba oil**—Ideal for both very dry and oily skin to help bring balance back. Use it with geranium, lavender and tea tree for tough skin conditions.

▶ **Magnesium oil**—Known as the ultimate relaxer. Blend it with Roman chamomile and lavender to reduce stress and improve sleep.

▶ **Arnica oil**—Best for treating bruises, pain and skin inflammation.

▶ **Shea butter**—The best carrier oil for moisturizing very dry and aged skin. It's also great for making a homemade body butter recipe.

▶ **Argan oil**—Known to firm and tighten skin, which is great for anti-aging effects. Mix it with frankincense, myrrh and geranium to improve skin tone. It's also packed with vitamin E.

▶ **Evening primrose oil**—Great for hormone balance because it contains high levels of GLA (gamma linoleic acid), which produces hormone-regulating prostaglandin. Mix it with clary sage, thyme and ylang ylang to support healthy hormones.

There are many other beneficial carrier oils such as olive, rosehip, hemp, sea buckthorn, black cumin, almond, apricot and pomegranate. For a more complete list of carrier oils, including their key benefits, please refer to Part II, which details individual essential and carrier oils.

When determining an appropriate topical dose, age and size are the biggest factors. The younger and smaller the person, the less essential oil is needed. *It is safest to start with a small amount and repeat the application 20 minutes later if necessary. In most cases, essential oils should be diluted with a carrier oil for use on the skin.*

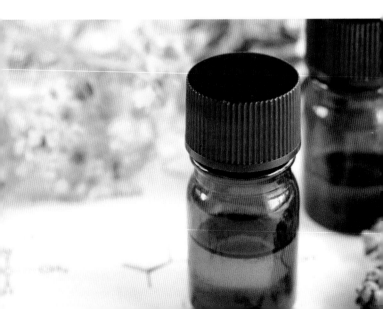

A generalized suggested ratio for dilution with a carrier oil is as follows:

For infants

1 drop of essential oil to 1 tablespoon carrier oil

For children

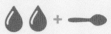

1 to 2 drops of essential oil to 1 teaspoon carrier oil

For adults

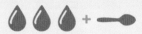

3 to 6 drops of essential oil to 1 teaspoon carrier oil

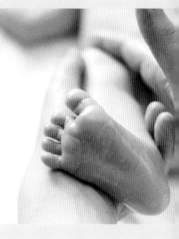

Once the essential oils are mixed with the carrier oil, rub the oils together in the palm with your fingers and apply the mixture to the specific area in circular, light massage movements.

Here are some other ways to use essential oils topically:

Baths. Adding oils to bath water is a mix of aromatic and topical applications. In order to disperse the oil throughout the bath water, add 5 to 15 drops of essential oils to bath salts or Epsom salts, which will dissolve in the water. This can help improve circulation, relieve sore muscles, soothe skin, open airways, relax the body and improve sleep. Soothing oils like eucalyptus and lavender are especially beneficial when added to an aromatherapy bath.

Compresses. Using a warm compress will increase the absorption of essential oils. Add 10 drops of oil per 4 ounces of water. Soak the cloth with the oil and water mixture and apply it to bruises, infections, aches and pains. (Peppermint is one of the best oils for muscle aches, while lavender is great for treating infections.)

Salves. A salve is an ointment that is used to soothe the surface of the body. You can make salves by adding 15 drops of essential oils to 1 ounce of a carrier oil (2.5 percent dilution). Salves can be stored in a metal or glass container and used on cuts, scrapes and sore muscles.

Personal Care. Essential oils can be used in common

home remedies like homemade toothpaste, deodorant, shampoo, conditioner, body wash, face wash, perfume, cologne, lip balm and body lotion. To make homemade teeth- and gum-supporting toothpaste, mix ¼ cup coconut oil, 3 tablespoons bentonite clay and 10 drops of peppermint or clove essential oil together and put the mixture into a rubber tube or sealed glass container.

TAKING ESSENTIAL OILS INTERNALLY

Essential oils are more potent than whole plant material. Remember that a single drop of rose oil contains the chemical constituents present in 60 roses. That is why when essential oils are used internally, it should be in small amounts only. However, research does show that many oils can be safe and effective when taken orally, so it may be worth the necessary preparation and caution for certain conditions and for short periods of time.

When an essential oil is consumed in high doses, it can result in overuse or toxicity. That is because essential oils are fat-soluble, meaning they are not easily eliminated from the body and must travel through the liver and then the gut. To avoid ingesting toxic concentrations of essential oils, labels should be read carefully and professional guidelines should be followed.

When we get the question, *"Are essential oils safe to use internally?"* our answer is always, "It depends upon which oil and the person taking the oil."

There is a sub-population of therapists who believe that essential oils should not be taken internally unless recommended by a physician. They recommend only topical or aromatic use. It's important to remember that a large amount of published articles and studies have demonstrated that many essential oils provide tremendous benefits when used internally, and traditional practitioners of Chinese and Ayurvedic medicine have used essential oils therapeutically for thousands of years.

It's all about using wisdom, applying common sense and remembering that following product usage directions is key in all supplement use—and when in doubt, use the oil topically. The three of us have personally used essential oils for ourselves and our families, clients and patients.

Some oils, like peppermint and lemon oil, can be consumed in small doses at 1 to 2 drops, two to three times a day. Other oils like oregano should only be consumed for a maximum of 10 days and under the guidance of a health care professional. Wintergreen should only be used topically or aromatically (diffused) and should never be used internally. People with liver disease and those who have higher levels of sensitivities need to be cautious. All essential oils should be taken with food or a beverage and not on an empty stomach.

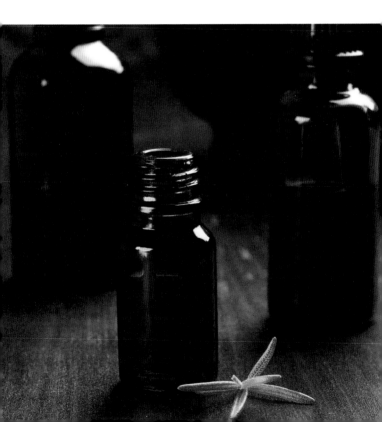

Suggested internal use methods for adults include:

Add 1 to 2 drops to a glass of water, almond milk or coconut milk

Put several drops of oil into an empty capsule and swallow with water

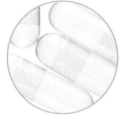

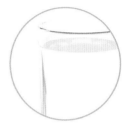

Add 1 to 2 drops to 1 teaspoon of raw honey and then consume

Add 1 to 2 drops to 1 teaspoon of coconut oil and then consume

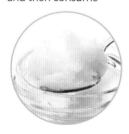

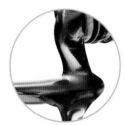

Drop certain oils directly under the tongue

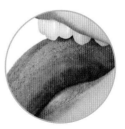

If you're someone who purchases and consumes organic foods, you should do your best to consume essential oil products that are certified organic.

When it comes to using oils on your body (topically) or taking them internally, safety is based on the properties of the oil itself, not the "quality" of the brand. *Some oils are simply not safe to take internally.* It is not wise to believe a company statement that asserts, "All of our oils are safe for internal use."

A bottle label may say "safe for supplemental use," but even then that doesn't necessarily mean it is safe when taken internally. *Some oils that are not safe for ingestion* include oils from the needles of trees such as pine essential oil and some bark oils such as cypress. Some essential oils are only suitable for external use because they have been linked to liver toxicity. These oils include aniseed, bay and tarragon.

Always consult with a doctor or healthcare practitioner before using essential oils internally. When in doubt, remember that with most essential oils, benefits can be found from topical and aromatherapy use.

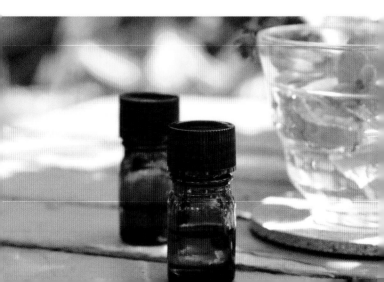

RESPECT THEIR POWER: OIL SIDE EFFECTS AND INTERACTIONS

A scientific review published by the *U.S National Library of Medicine* in 2014 states that safety testing on essential oils shows very few negative side effects or risks when they are used as directed. Some essential oils have been approved as ingredients in food and are classified as GRAS (generally recognized as safe) by the U.S. Food and Drug Administration, within specific limits.

However, like all medicine, they are not without their risks and possible complications.

It takes a small amount of essential oils to prompt a powerful therapeutic benefit. Because essential oils are so concentrated, they must be used with care. Labels should be read carefully and guidelines followed vigilantly. *Essential oils should never be applied to the eyes or ear canals.* After handling essential oils, avoid accidental eye contact by washing your hands. If essential oils get into the eye, place a few drops of a carrier oil in the eye and blink until the oil clears out.

If you are taking prescription or over-the-counter (OTC) medications, be aware that using an essential oil along with a drug can increase the drug's side effects. The chemical constituents of the essential oil could inhibit the drug's metabolizing enzymes, rendering the drug unable to be excreted or metabolized properly. Grapefruit essential oil specifically has been shown to interfere with medications.

Before using essential oils, research the oil's drug interactions or speak to a health care provider about possible outcomes. For example, people who are taking heart medications, such as blood thinners, should avoid using clary sage, cypress, eucalyptus, ginger, rosemary, sage and thyme oils.

The International Fragrance Association has banned several essential oils because they are toxic when ingested or applied topically. These oils include cade oil crude, costus root, elecampane, fig leaf absolute, horseradish, nightshade, pennyroyal, rue, sassafras, savin, southernwood, stinging nettle, stryax gum, tea absolute, wormseed and wormwood.

Allergic reactions and skin irritation may occur, especially when essential oils are in contact with the skin for long periods of time. In fact, sun sensitivity may develop when citrus or other oils are applied to the skin before sun exposure.

Finally, lavender and tea tree oils have been found to have hormone-like effects similar to estrogen. On the other hand, many studies, including one published in *Evidence Based Complementary Alternative Medicine* concludes that lavender oil effectively relieves stress, anxiety, depression, neurological conditions and cognitive conditions.[18] Lavender oil and tea tree oil are known to reduce pain and work as antioxidants and anti-inflammatory agents. Some essential oils that are better for regulating hormone levels include Roman chamomile, sandalwood and clary sage.

Keep in mind that **essential oils are highly concentrated substances**. One drop is powerful enough to soothe sore muscles, relieve an itchy bug bite or stop a cold in its tracks. Don't be fooled by their "natural" origin. Their power must be respected—they have the potential to cause minor reactions, such as skin irritation, or more serious consequences like respiratory failure, when not used appropriately.

Before experimenting with an oil, become familiar with its properties, dosage instructions and precautions. When in

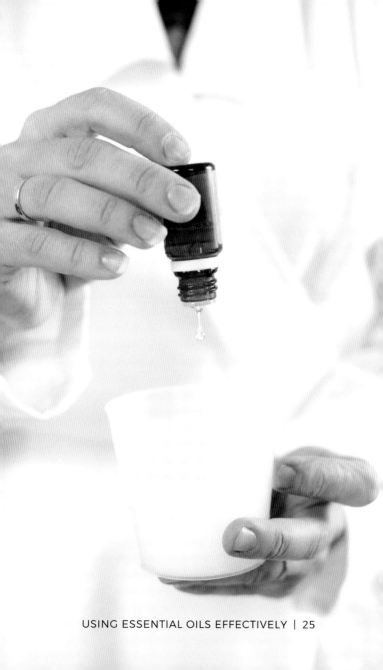

doubt about a condition or an oil, consult a qualified medical specialist. There is no regulated standard, which means it is up to users to educate themselves on the proper use of each essential oil before using them.

CINNAMON BARK

CINNAMOMUM VERUM

As early as 2000 B.C., Egyptians employed cinnamon and cassia as perfuming agents during the embalming process, and cinnamon was even mentioned in the Old Testament as an ingredient in the holy anointing oil. Legend also has it that the Roman emperor Nero burned as much as he could find of the precious spice on the funeral pyre of his second wife Poppaea Sabina in A.D. 65 to atone for his role in her death.

Cinnamon bark oil is extracted by steam distillation from the outer bark of the cinnamon tree and has been touted for its medicinal properties for thousands of years. The warm and intense aroma of cinnamon bark can stimulate the appetite and ignite the senses. Cinnamon bark oil is highly concentrated with antioxidants, which makes it effective as a natural digestive aid, blood sugar stabilizer and circulation booster. It's also commonly used to combat cardiovascular diseases and to aid in fighting infections.

SUPER 7 RX

1. Boosts Heart Health

Because of its circulation-boosting abilities, cinnamon oil can support the cleansing of arteries. Apply 2 to 3 drops of cinnamon oil mixed with ½ teaspoon of coconut oil to your chest to promote warmth and increased blood flow.

2. Supports Healthy Blood Sugar and Insulin Release

Cinnamon oil may help keep blood sugar stable and prevent chronic fatigue, moodiness, sugar cravings and overeating. Inhale cinnamon essential oil, diffuse it or apply it to your chest and wrists.

3. May Help with High Cholesterol

One study revealed that a key constituent in cinnamon bark oil, cinnamate, lowers the activity of an enzyme that makes cholesterol in the body called HMG CoA reductase—the same enzyme targeted by statins. Take 1 to 2 drops of cinnamon essential oil internally to fight high cholesterol.

4. Helps Fight Infections

Diffusing cinnamon bark essentialoil has shown an inhibitory effect against respiratory tract pathogens, including some penicillin-resistant strains. Diffuse it daily for protection against infection or to relieve a present infection.

CINNAMON BARK USES

5. Promotes Weight Loss

Because cinnamon oil can balance blood sugar levels
and improve the taste of foods without added sugar, it's
effective for curbing a sweet tooth. Add 1 to 2 drops to
fruit, oats, baked goods or smoothies to help slow the
rate at which glucose is released into the blood.

6. Fights Parasites

Studies have found that cinnamon oil inhibits the
growth of certain harmful parasites. Ingest the oil to
fight harmful parasites and impede parasite growth.

7. Soothes Sore Throat

Cinnamon oil can help prevent mucus buildup and clear
nasal passages. Drink hot lemon water, honey and 1 drop
of cinnamon oil in the morning to soothe a sore throat
(plus curb cravings and support immune function).

RESEARCH STUDIES

A 2011 study found that a 70 percent methanolic extract of cinnamon oil showed significant ability to enhance immune function by combatting oxidative stress.[1]

A 2012 study concluded that *Cinnamomum verum* volatile oil applied either separately or in combination with other oil extracts had the most effective anti-microbial activity against certain infectious diseases.[2]

 ## KEY BENEFITS

- Helps decrease inflammation
- Increases circulation
- Contains anti-viral properties
- Fights free radicals
- May help relieve depression
- Stimulates the immune system
- Boosts libido
- Fights parasites

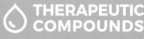 ## THERAPEUTIC COMPOUNDS

Cinnamaldehyde Eugenol

Methyleugenol Phellandrene

 ## SAFETY

People with sensitive skin may experience skin irritation when using cinnamon oil topically or internally. Test a small amount first, mixed with a carrier oil.

CLARY SAGE

SALVIA SCLAREA

Clary sage has a surprising and fascinating history. Medieval authors called the herb "clear eye" and considered it beneficial in healing visual problems. In fact, "clary" is derived from the Latin word "clarus," which means clear. In the Middle Ages, it was known as "Oculus Christi," or the "eyes of Christ." In Chinese medicine, sage is used to strengthen the kidneys, adrenals and female reproductive organs. Clary sage is considered one of the top essential oils for balancing hormones, especially in women. It is highly beneficial when dealing with cramps, heavy menstrual cycles, hot flashes and hormonal imbalances.

The flower from the clary sage plant is steam-distilled, and it has a musky but feminine and balancing aroma. The main chemical component of clary sage oil is linalyl acetate, making it one of the most relaxing, soothing and balancing essential oils. Inhaling clary sage oil may promote feelings of relaxation, allowing for a restful night's sleep. It's also known for its ability to support healthy circulation, digestion and eye health.

SUPER 7 RX

1. Supports Hormonal Balance

Clary sage oil contains natural phytoestrogens, which give it the ability to produce estrogenic effects. The oil can help regulate estrogen levels and support the long-term health of the uterus. To help balance hormones, apply 3 drops regularly to your abdomen, 2 drops to your neck or diffuse the oil.

2. Helps with Menstrual Discomfort

Clary sage oil has the power to alleviate some of the symptoms of PMS. It is also anti-spasmodic, meaning it can treat spasms and muscle cramps. To relieve menstrual discomfort, take it internally or apply it topically to your abdomen.

3. Promotes Restfulness

Clary sage oil is a natural sedative. To help relieve insomnia and feelings of anxiety, diffuse it at your bedside or rub 1 to 2 drops onto your neck and the soles of your feet.

4. Supports Healthy Circulation

By opening up the blood vessels and allowing for increased blood circulation, clary sage oil may be beneficial to the heart. It also naturally lowers blood pressure by relaxing the brain and arteries. Rub the oil onto your limbs and chest.

CLARY SAGE USES

5. May Help Lower Cholesterol

The anti-inflammatory and antioxidant properties of clary sage oil may help to lower cholesterol naturally. Diffuse it or add 5 drops to a warm-water bath.

6. Contains Compounds Beneficial for Fighting Leukemia

A chemical compound found in clary sage oil, called sclareol, is able to kill leukemia cell lines through apoptosis. An insufficient amount of apoptosis results in uncontrolled abnormal cell proliferation, i.e. cancer. Take clary sage oil internally to promote apoptosis.

7. Boosts Skin Health

An important ester in clary sage oil, called linalyl acetate, has been shown to reduce skin inflammation and work as a natural remedy for rashes. Combine clary sage oil with jojoba oil and apply it to your skin.

RESEARCH STUDIES

Evidence suggests that aromatherapy can be effective in reducing maternal anxiety, fear and pain during labor. Of the essential oils that were tested, clary sage oil and Roman chamomile oil were the most effective in alleviating pain.[3]

Results of a 2015 study support the use of formulations containing clary sage oil as the active natural anti-microbial agent. Because of its anti-microbial properties, clary sage oil may be applied to wounds and skin infections.[4]

✓ KEY BENEFITS

- Supports hormone balance
- May increase circulation
- Can improve mood
- Helps reduce stress
- Contains anti-fungal and antiseptic properties
- May relieve asthma symptoms
- Boosts eye, hair and skin health

THERAPEUTIC COMPOUNDS

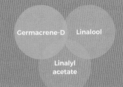

Germacrene-D Linalool

Linalyl acetate

✓ SAFETY

Clary sage oil is not safe for use during pregnancy, especially during the first trimester or when using it on the abdomen, because it can cause uterine contractions.

EUCALYPTUS

EUCALYPTUS RADIATA

According to English folklore, an early English settler had his thumb nearly severed by an ax. His father, who was well versed in Aboriginal folk medicine, advised that he apply a bandage of tightly bound eucalyptus leaves around the cut after it was sutured. Later, when a surgeon saw the wound, he remarked how amazed he was because the thumb healed so quickly and without any trace of infection.

The eucalyptus tree (also known as Tasmanian Blue Gum) is an evergreen tree native to Australia that's often thought of as the main food source of koala bears. While it provides amazing nutritional support for wildlife, the essential oil that is extracted from eucalyptus leaves also has powerful therapeutic properties. Eucalyptus has a cool, crisp aroma. The main chemical components of *Eucalyptus radiata* are eucalyptol and alpha-terpineol, making it an ideal oil to promote feelings of clear breathing and open airways and for creating a soothing massage experience.

SUPER 7 RX

1. Helps Ease Symptoms of Bronchitis and Pneumonia

Eucalyptus can ease symptoms of respiratory conditions by dilating the blood vessels and allowing more oxygen into the lungs. Mix 3 to 5 drops with equal parts of peppermint and coconut oil to make a homemade vapor rub; rub the mixture onto your chest.

2. Reduces Earaches

Eucalyptus can be an effective treatment for earaches. Add several drops of eucalyptus oil to a pan of boiling water, remove the pan from the heat, place a towel over your head and inhale the steam. Also try gently massaging the oil into the skin around your ear.

3. Helps Improve Asthma and Allergies

Studies show that eucalyptus oil is effective at treating sinusitis and that patients sometimes experience faster improvement when using the oil for allergies, breathing and sinus issues. Gargle with 1 to 2 drops of eucalyptus oil or apply it topically to your chest.

4. Promotes Energy and Focus

To feel energized, alert and focused,diffuse eucalyptus throughout your home or at work, or rub a few drops on your temples or neck.

EUCALYPTUS USES

5. Provides Relief from Shingles

Eucalyptus oil may help with the pain associated with shingles. Apply eucalyptus to your skin for instant relief from itching and pain.

6. Serves as a Cleaning Aid

Because of its anti-microbial properties, eucalyptus oil can help disinfect the home. Put 10 to 15 drops into home-care products such as laundry detergent and toilet cleaner. It can also be added to vacuums or a diffuser to inhibit the growth of mold and bacteria in the home.

7. Aids in Wound Care

Because of its anti-microbial and antiseptic properties, eucalyptus oil effectively treats wounds, burns, cuts, insect stings, abrasions, sores and scrapes. It also fights infections and may speed healing. Apply eucalyptus oil to the affected area twice daily.

RESEARCH STUDIES

Eucalyptus oil has been found to be effective in reducing pain, swelling and inflammation. When used on patients who underwent a total knee replacement, eucalyptus inhalation significantly lowered blood pressure and pain levels.[5]

A 2015 research study concluded that topical application of 1,8-cineole (the primary active ingredient in eucalyptus) offers a novel therapeutic approach to reduce infection-induced mucus secretion.[6]

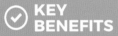 KEY BENEFITS

- Reduces earaches
- May reduce fever
- Fights infections
- Boosts mental clarity
- Relieves respiratory conditions
- Helps reduce pain and inflammation
- Aids in disinfecting house and clothes
- Serves as a remedy for skin irritations and insect bites

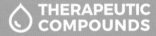 THERAPEUTIC COMPOUNDS

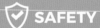

Alpha-Terpineol

Eucalyptol (1,8-cineole)

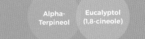 SAFETY

People with sensitive skin should dilute eucalyptus oil before topical use. Also, dilute it before using with children. Do not apply near the face of young children.

FRANKINCENSE

BOSWELLIA FREREANA, BOSWELLIA CARTERII, BOSWELLIA SACRA

Often called the "king of oils," frankincense is powerful, effective and incredibly therapeutic. For thousands of years, religious followers have used frankincense during worship, meditation and spiritual practices. The word frankincense appears 17 times in the Bible, and the word incense is mentioned 113 times; in such cases, incense is often assumed to imply frankincense along with myrrh and other spices. A beautiful small tree or shrub with abundant pinnate leaves and white or pale pink flowers, frankincense yields a natural oleo gum resin that is collected by making incisions into the bark. Its essential oil is collected from the resin through steam distillation.

One of the most prized and precious essential oils, frankincense has extraordinary health benefits. It is used to help relieve chronic stress and anxiety, reduce pain and inflammation, boost immunity and even combat tumors. The sesquiterpenes in frankincense enable it to go beyond the blood-brain barrier. It also increases the activity of leukocytes, which help the body fight infections. We wonder if the magi from the East knew of frankincense's healing properties when they presented it to young Jesus?

SUPER 7 RX

1. Serves as a Powerful Addition to Cancer-Fighting Protocols

Frankincense essential oil has been shown to help fight specific types of cancer cells. Take 2 to 3 drops internally, use as a suppository (under the supervision of a health practitioner) or massage the oil onto the affected area to support healthy immune system response.

2. May Relieve Joint Inflammation and Pain

To improve circulation and help relieve symptoms of joint or muscle pain related to conditions such as arthritis, digestive disorders and asthma, massage frankincense oil onto the painful area or diffuse.

3. Boosts the Immune System

Studies have demonstrated that frankincense has immune-enhancing abilities. It can be used to prevent germs from forming on the skin, in the mouth or in the home. Diffuse it, take it internally or rub onto your temples, wrists and the soles of your feet.

4. Promotes Relaxation During Meditation and Prayer

Frankincense oil may help induce a feeling of peace and relaxation, making it ideal for prayer time and meditation. Diffuse it during meditation and anoint your family with this ancient, powerful oil.

FRANKINCENSE USES

5. Relieves Cold and Flu Symptoms

Frankincense oil can help eliminate phlegm in the lungs and acts as an anti-inflammatory agent in the nasal passages. To treat respiratory conditions, add 5 drops of frankincense oil to a diffuser and breathe in deeply for 5 minutes, or rub 2 to 3 drops onto your chest.

6. Reduces the Appearance of Stretch Marks and Wrinkles

Frankincense oil can help minimize stretch marks, scars and wrinkles. Mix 2 to 3 drops of the oil with equal parts of coconut or jojoba oil and apply to the affected areas.

7. Helps Those with Brain Injury and Alzheimer's

Because it improves cognitive health and responses, frankincense oil may be used on people with Alzheimer's disease, dementia and brain injury. Take it internally, diffuse it, or apply it topically to the back of your neck and under your nose.

RESEARCH STUDIES

Frankincense oil has been shown to induce breast cancer cell death, suggesting that it is effective against breast cancer. Frankincense represses signaling pathways and cell cycle regulators that have been proposed as therapeutic targets for breast cancer.[7]

A 2011 study found that frankincense essential oil has anti-inflammatory effects in the treatment of gingivitis. After frankincense treatment, participants showed significant decreases in gingivitis index, plaque index and probing pocket depth.[8]

 ## KEY BENEFITS

- Combats negative emotions and stress
- Supports immunity and helps prevent illness
- Contains anti-tumor properties
- Heightens spiritual awareness
- Lessens the signs of aging skin
- Encourages healthy hormone levels
- May ease digestion
- Helps relieve inflammation and pain

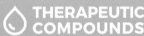 ## THERAPEUTIC COMPOUNDS

Alpha-Pinene

Alpha-Thujene

Limonene

 ## SAFETY

Frankincense is known to have blood-thinning effects, so people with problems related to blood clotting should not use before consulting with their health care provider.

LAVENDER

LAVANDULA ANGUSTIFOLIA

Ancient texts tell us that lavender has been used for medicinal and religious purposes for over 2,500 years. The Egyptians used it for mummification and as perfume. The Romans used it for cooking and scenting the air. They also added lavender to their bath water, hence the name from the Latin "lavare" meaning "to wash."

In quite possibly the most famous usage of all, Mary may have applied lavender with her hair to anoint Jesus. Interestingly, many researchers claim that 2,000 years ago lavender was referred to as spikenard or simply "nard" from the Greek name for lavender, naardus, after the Syrian city of Naarda. According to John 12:3, "Mary then took a pound of very costly perfume of pure nard, and anointed the feet of Jesus and wiped His feet with her hair; and the house was filled with the fragrance of the perfume."

Today, lavender oil is the most commonly used essential oil in the world. It is often considered a "must-have" oil to keep on hand at all times due to its versatile uses, including relaxing properties that promote peaceful sleep and ease feelings of tension. The lavender flowers are steam-distilled for their essential oil, and the aroma is floral, sweet and calming.

SUPER 7 RX

1. Promotes Sleep

To help get a good night's rest, diffuse 5 drops of lavender oil beside your bed, or apply 2 to 3 drops to the back of your neck, as well as your chest and temples.

2. Soothes Burns, Sunburns and Cuts

Lavender has been shown to be highly soothing to skin cuts and irritations. Mix lavender oil with coconut oil and apply it to the areas of concern twice daily.

3. Helps Relieve Anxiety and Stress

Lavender oil is known to bring on feelings of peace and relaxation. Diffuse lavender oil, add it to a warm-water bath or apply it to your temples, wrists and the soles of your feet.

4. Combats High Blood Pressure

Diffuse lavender oil beside you during your workday to help soothe stressed behaviors and promote healthy blood pressure.

LAVENDER USES

5. Stimulates Healthy Blood Sugar Balance

Lavender oil shows promise in protecting the body from increases in blood glucose. Apply it to the back of your neck and your chest, diffuse it or add 1 drop to a glass of water or cup of tea.

6. Helps Relieve Headaches and Migraines

For relief from headache pain, inhale lavender oil for 15 minutes. You can also mix 2 drops of lavender oil with 2 drops of peppermint oil and apply it to the back of your neck and your temples for a tension and pain relief aid.

7. Encourages Healthy Skin

Lavender oil can be applied directly on the skin or mixed with coconut oil for those with sensitivities. Mixing lavender oil with equal parts frankincense oil will help boost skin health.

RESEARCH STUDIES

A 2014 study found lavender oil not only lessened the severity of lab-induced diabetes, but also improved body weight and protected the liver and kidneys from degeneration in laboratory animals.[9]

A 2013 study found that taking 80 milligrams of lavender essential oil internally via capsules alleviated insomnia, anxiety and depression, and also improved Alzheimer's symptoms. Another study found that lavender oil reduced depression by 32.7 percent in people suffering from post-traumatic stress disorder (PTSD).[10] [11]

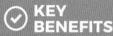

KEY BENEFITS

- Helps improve sleep
- May reduce anxiety and depression
- Serves as first aid for burns and wounds
- Improves skin and reduces acne
- Proves helpful for eczema and psoriasis
- Helps relieve headaches
- Promotes balanced blood sugar
- Helps lower blood pressure

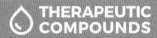

THERAPEUTIC COMPOUNDS

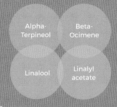

Alpha-Terpineol

Beta-Ocimene

Linalool

Linalyl acetate

SAFETY

For most people, lavender oil is well tolerated.

LEMON

CITRUS LIMON

Ayurvedic medicine practitioners have been using lemon essential oil to treat a wide spectrum of health conditions for at least 1,000 years. In Traditional Chinese Medicine, lemon peel oil has the ability to combat conditions related to dampness such as the common cold, candida, infections, loose stools, respiratory conditions and sore throats. Also, it has been used throughout history to support the health of the liver and as a natural remedy for gallstones. Lemon oil contains the compound d-limonene, which also has powerful anti-cancer properties.

Lemon oil is known for its ability to help cleanse toxins from any part of the body; it is widely used to stimulate lymph drainage, rejuvenate energy, purify skin and repel insects. The rind of the lemon is cold-pressed for the extraction of its essential oil, which has a sweet, citrusy and sharp aroma that is uplifting and refreshing. Lemon is a powerful cleansing agent that purifies the air and surfaces, and it can be used as a non-toxic cleaner throughout the home. When added to water, lemon oil provides a refreshing and healthy boost throughout the day.

SUPER 7 RX

1. Promotes Lymphatic Drainage

Lemon oil is beneficial for improving blood flow and reducing swelling in lymph nodes. Apply 1 to 2 drops topically directly to your lymph nodes or diffuse it.

2. Helps Clear Mucus and Phlegm

Lemon oil helps to relieve congestion and eliminate mucus. It can also slow a runny nose and reduce the symptoms of allergies. Inhale lemon oil directly from the bottle or apply it topically, mixed with a carrier oil, to your chest and nose.

3. May Improve Mood

Help lift mood, improve concentration, fight depression and combat addiction by diffusing lemon essential oil, or apply it topically to your wrists and chest.

4. Assists in Gallbladder Health and Gallstone Removal

To help pass painful gallstones, mix 1 quart of sauerkraut juice, 1 quart of tomato juice, 10 drops of lemon oil and 10 drops of peppermint oil. Divide the mixture into two jars. Drink one jar the first morning, and the second jar the following morning.

LEMON USES

5. Boosts the Immune System

Lemon essential oil has anti-bacterial properties, and it helps the body get rid of toxins that could lead to illness. Research shows that lemon oil protects the body against human pathogens such as E. coli and salmonella. To boost the immune system, take it internally.

6. Proves Effective for Cleaning Multiple Surfaces

Disinfect and degrease your home, car or office with lemon oil. Add it to a spray bottle of water to clean tables, countertops and other surfaces. Lemon oil also makes a great furniture polish; simply add a few drops to olive oil to clean, protect and shine wood.

7. Lessens Allergy Symptoms

Lemon oil can help to combat seasonal allergies and asthma attacks. It works as a natural antihistamine, relieves excess mucus and cools down inflammation. Take 1 to 2 drops internally mixed with equal parts of peppermint and lavender for allergy relief.

RESEARCH STUDIES

A 2014 study found that lemon oil aromatherapy reduced nausea and vomiting during pregnancy. The nausea and vomiting intensity in the lemon oil group were significantly lower than the control group.[12]

Lemon essential oil has proven strong anti-stress effects. In a study, mice were exposed to three behavioral tasks. After utilizing lemon oil, the results suggested that it possessed notable antidepressant-like effects on the mice during these tasks.[13]

KEY BENEFITS

- Helps purify the body
- Freshens breath
- Aids in cough suppression
- Supports fat digestion
- Fights cancer
- Stimulates lymphatic drainage
- Promotes weight loss

THERAPEUTIC COMPOUNDS

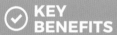

Alpha-Pinenes

Beta-Pinenes

D-Limonene

SAFETY

Avoid direct sunlight for up to 12 hours after external application.

MELALEUCA
(TEA TREE)

MELALEUCA ALTERNIFOLIA

Melaleuca, or tea tree oil, has been passed down for thousands of years by the native indigenous Bundjalung aborigines of Australia. While their healers tended to use spiritual medicine to heal serious illnesses, they also used the leaves of the tea tree plant to treat more common medical concerns. As legend has it, there was one "mystical" lake where the tea tree leaves had been falling for hundreds of years and that the mud became saturated with the tea tree oil. This mud was applied to skin for medicinal purposes.

Melaleuca essential oil is well known for its powerful antiseptic properties and ability to treat wounds. For over 70 years, tea tree oil has been documented in numerous medical studies for its ability to kill many strains of bacteria, viruses and fungi. The leaves of the melaleuca plant are steam-distilled to extract the essential oil. Tea tree has a fresh, woody, earthy and medicinal aroma that has powerful cleansing and purifying properties. The Earth is rich with natural healing power, and there may be no better example of this than melaleuca. It purifies as it heals and is a must for any home medicine cabinet.

SUPER 7 RX

1. Treats Acne

Tea tree oil is considered one of the most effective home treatments for acne. It is reportedly just as effective as benzoyl peroxide but without the associated negative side effects that many people experience. Create a gentle and effective face wash by mixing 5 drops of tea tree oil with 2 teaspoons of raw honey.

2. Helps with Dandruff

Tea tree oil soothes dry, flaking skin and can be used as a natural treatment for head lice. Add 5 drops of tea tree oil to shampoo or conditioner, or make a natural shampoo by combining 5 to 10 drops of tea tree oil with aloe vera gel, coconut milk and lavender oil.

3. Disinfects the Home

Tea tree oil has powerful anti-microbial properties, allowing it to fight bad bacteria in the home. Combine tea tree oil with water, vinegar and lemon essential oil, and add it to a spray bottle to use on countertops, kitchen appliances, showers, toilets and sinks.

4. Helps Treat Psoriasis and Eczema

Use tea tree oil to relieve skin inflammation associated with conditions such as psoriasis and eczema. Make an anti-inflammatory and soothing lotion by combining 5 drops of tea tree oil, 5 drops of lavender oil and 1 teaspoon of coconut oil. Apply it topically twice daily.

5. May Remedy Toenail Fungus and Ringworm

Because of its ability to kill fungi, tea tree oil is a great choice to use on toenail fungus, athlete's foot and ringworm. Apply it topically to the affected area. For stubborn fungi, mix tea tree with oregano oil.

6. Acts as a Natural Deodorant

Because of its anti-microbial properties, tea tree oil can destroy the bacteria on the skin that causes body odor. Combine 5 drops of tea tree oil with 1 teaspoon each of coconut oil and baking soda. Apply the mixture to your armpits or even in your shoes or sports gear.

7. Cleans Infections and Cuts

The antiseptic and anti-bacterial properties of tea tree oil make it a natural treatment for cuts, wounds, burns and skin infections or irritations. Combine 2 drops of tea tree oil with 2 drops of lavender oil, and apply it directly to the area of concern.

RESEARCH STUDIES

A 2007 study used a 5 percent tea tree oil topical gel to treat acne lesions. The results found that those who used tea tree oil had approximately a 5-times greater improvement in acne than those who did not use the treatment.[14]

Tea tree oil was found to inhibit 301 different types of yeast isolated from the mouths of patients, demonstrating the effectiveness of using tea tree oil in treating oral yeast in cancer patients and the use in oral hygiene products.[15]

KEY BENEFITS

- Treats acne
- Helps treat chickenpox
- Provides relief for cold sores
- Can ease earaches
- Serves as a remedy for bad breath
- Prevents and helps kill head lice
- Works as a natural deodorant
- Inhibits mold growth

THERAPEUTIC COMPOUNDS

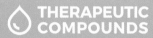

Alpha- & Y-Terpinenes

Terpinen-4-ol

P-Cymene

SAFETY

Melaleuca (tea tree) oil should not be taken internally for any reason. If using tea tree in the mouth (as in a mouthwash or toothpaste), spit out the oil afterwards to prevent potential side effects such as digestive issues, hives or dizziness.

MYRRH

COMMIPHORA MYRRHA

Discovered more than 3,700 years ago, myrrh was used by the Ancient Egyptians during the embalming process and in perfumes and cosmetics. Ancient records show that myrrh was deemed so valuable that at times it was valued at its weight in gold. Myrrh essential oil is well known because it was mentioned 152 times in the Bible, serving as a spice, natural remedy, means to purify the dead and, of course, as a gift from the magi to baby Jesus.

Myrrh essential oil has potent antioxidant activity and has been researched as a potential cancer treatment. The resin of the myrrh tree is dried and steam-distilled; the essential oil has a smoky, sweet and sometimes bitter aroma. An ancient healer and treatment for a multitude of ailments and symptoms, myrrh is a remarkable essential oil that you will likely run out of quickly.

SUPER 7 RX

1. Acts as an Anti-inflammatory

Myrrh has healing, anti-bacterial, anti-fungal and anti-inflammatory properties that may reduce swelling and treat infections. Add 2 to 3 drops of myrrh oil to a cold compress and apply it directly to the infected or inflamed area.

2.Promotes Awareness During Prayer and Meditation

Because of its significance in the Bible, using myrrh is ideal during prayer and meditation. Diffuse it to help promote awareness and connect with God during meditation, and anoint others with the oil.

3. Helps Treats Vaginal and Oral Yeast

To treat Candida overgrowth, take 1 drop of myrrh oil internally, or dilute 2 to 3 drops with equal parts of a carrier oil and apply it topically to affected areas. For oral thrush, add 1 to 2 drops to natural mouthwash and gargle several times a day.

4. May Alleviate Gum Disease and Mouth Infections

Myrrh oil may help to relieve inflammation of the mouth and gums caused by diseases such as gingivitis and mouth ulcers. Add to mouthwash or toothpaste to help prevent gum disease and mouth infections.

MYRRH USES

5. Fights Parasites and Fungal Infections

Myrrh is a natural treatment for parasites, and it can also help to reduce fungal infections such as athlete's foot or ringworm. To fight infection, take 1 to 2 drops internally with water or in a capsule, or apply it directly to the fungal infection site.

6. Displays Cancer-Fighting Qualities

Myrrh is being studied for its potential anti-cancer benefits. Apply it directly to a skin cancer site twice daily. Myrrh oil is also an astringent, so it strengthens the body's cells, helps to stop bleeding and may prevent hair loss by strengthening hair roots.

7. Treats Wounds and Ulcers

Myrrh oil has the power to increase the function of white blood cells, which are critical for wound healing. It can decrease the incidence of ulcers and improve their healing time. Apply 2 to 3 drops, diluted with a carrier oil, to the affected area twice daily.

RESEARCH STUDIES

A 2013 study reported the anti-cancer effects of myrrh essential oil. The cell death rate was higher in the myrrh essential oil group compared with that of the other tested groups, including frankincense. The results also indicated that breast cancer cells exhibited increased sensitivity to myrrh oil.[16]

A study identifies myrrh oil as an anti-inflammatory and wound-healing product. Treatment with myrrh induced an initial increase in white blood cell levels that persisted through the post-injury healing period.[17]

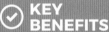

KEY BENEFITS

- Has anti-cancer properties
- Serves as a potent antioxidant
- Contains anti-bacterial and anti-fungal properties
- Fights parasites
- Boosts skin health
- Aids relaxation
- Helps relieve congestion
- Can fight infections and support wound healing

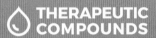

THERAPEUTIC COMPOUNDS

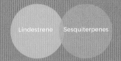

Lindestrene   Sesquiterpenes

SAFETY

Do not use it during pregnancy, as myrrh oil is fetotoxic (poisonous to a fetus). Myrrh oil may lower blood sugar levels, so it is not recommended for people with diabetes or other blood sugar conditions. For topical use, dilute it with a carrier oil and test it on a small area.

ORANGE

CITRUS SINENSIS

Orange (often known as sweet orange) has a fascinating historical and even mythical background. The Japanese believed citrus blossoms represented chastity. Ancient Arab women used it to color gray hair. Nostradamus wrote about how to use its blossoms and fruit to make cosmetics. Hercules so valued it that he stole the golden fruit from Hesperides, who protected it as the primary food of the ancient Roman and Greek gods.

Interestingly, sweet orange does not occur as a wild plant anywhere in the world, and is thought to be a natural hybrid of the pummelo *(Citrus maxima)* and the mandarin *(Citrus reticulata)*. Orange essential oil is cold-pressed from the outer peel of the common orange fruit. It is used for its anti-cancer, antidepressant, digestive and sedative properties. Possessing a citrusy and tart aroma, orange oil uplifts your emotions while sweeping away stress. It can also work as a secret weapon in the kitchen against stubborn grease stains.

SUPER 7 RX

1. Provides Immune System Support

Orange oil has virus- and bacteria-fighting abilities. To boost the immune system and fight free radical damage, take 1 to 2 drops of orange oil internally. Place it under your tongue or add it to a glass of water or your favorite beverage.

2. Displays Cancer-Fighting Properties

The anti-cancer activity of orange oil is largely due to the presence of limonene. There are now over 200 research articles on limonene, supporting its effective chemo-preventive agents against cancer cells. Put 1 to 2 drops of orange oil into your favorite tea, juice or sparkling water.

3. Encourages Lymphatic Drainage

Orange oil may stimulate the lymphatic system, liver, kidneys and bladder—drawing out toxins, excess sodium and waste from the digestive tract. Dilute 2 to 4 drops of orange oil with coconut oil and gently rub it onto your lymph nodes, chest and lymphatic pathways.

4. Fights Anxiety

Orange essential oil is an anxiety-reducing oil thanks to its calming properties. Diffusing orange oil, adding some to your body wash or inhaling it directly may fight anxiety and lower stress levels.

ORANGE USES

5. Improves Mood

Orange oil has a direct effect on the brain's olfactory system that quickly evokes emotional responses—lifting moods and promoting relaxation. Diffuse orange oil or apply it topically.

6. Boosts Digestion

As an anti-inflammatory agent, relaxant and circulation-enhancer, orange oil promotes better digestion and may help ease cramps or constipation. Apply 2 to 3 drops to your abdominal area to boost digestion. To improve detoxification, take 1 to 2 drops internally; this encourages an increase in urine production and may prevent bloating.

7. Serves as a Natural Household Cleaner

Orange oil has a fresh and citrusy smell, and it has the power to fight bacteria and microorganisms in your home. Add orange oil to a spray bottle filled with water and use it on countertops, appliances, showers, toilets and sinks.

RESEARCH STUDIES

A 2010 study found that orange oil could effectively help stop the growth of human lung and colon cancer cells. This is due to orange oil's PMFs (flavonoid antioxidants) that have been shown to halt cancer proliferation and trigger cancer cell death.[18]

A recent study showed that orange and rose essential oil may relax the brain. After half of a test group was exposed to diffused orange and rose oil for 90 seconds, they experienced notable increases in "comfortable," "relaxed" and "natural" feelings.[19]

 ## KEY BENEFITS

- Eases cold and flu symptoms
- Demonstrates anti-tumor activity
- Helps reduce appearance of wrinkles
- Acts as a natural anti-bacterial agent
- Aids in easing anxiety
- May increase circulation
- May improve blood pressure
- Supports lymphatic drainage

THERAPEUTIC COMPOUNDS

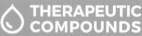

Limonene   Myrcene

 ## SAFETY

Avoid direct sunlight for up to 12 hours after external application. Orange oil can cause reactions on sensitive skin, so test on a small area first.

OREGANO

ORIGANUM VULGARE

Oregano has been a precious commodity for over 2,500 years and a popular folk medicine remedy. Hippocrates, the ancient Greek physician and the father of Western medicine, used oregano as an antiseptic for treating respiratory and digestive diseases. Ancient Greeks believed oregano was a useful poison antidote and used it extensively to treat skin infections, sore throats, wounds and viral infections. Traditional Chinese Medicine practitioners have also used oregano for generations to treat diarrhea, parasites and fungal infections.

The oregano plant is known for its potent flavor, as well as its therapeutic properties. The oregano leaves are steam-distilled, and the essential oil has a sharp and herbaceous aroma. Oregano essential oil is an incredible natural antibiotic because it contains carvacrol and thymol, two powerful compounds with anti-bacterial and anti-fungal properties. Dozens of studies confirm that oregano oil can be used along with or as an alternative to antibiotics for a number of health concerns. The research supports the fact that oregano is more than just an antibiotic—it's the *ultimate* natural antibiotic!

SUPER 7 RX

1. Acts as a Natural Antibiotic

Oregano oil has anti-bacterial properties that are powerful enough to kill different types of bad bacteria, including E. Coli. It can prevent bacterial overgrowth and colonization in the large intestine, and it helps protect the body from toxicity. Dilute it with a carrier oil and apply it topically to the soles of your feet or take it internally for 10 days at a time and then cycle off.

2. Battles Candida and Fungal Overgrowth

Oil of oregano can be used to treat fungi and yeast such as candida. Oregano can also treat toenail fungus when used topically. For internal use, take 2 to 4 drops twice daily for up to 10 days.

3. Helps Fight Pneumonia and Bronchitis

Oregano oil can help prevent or fight pneumonia, bronchitis and other types of bacterial infections. For external infections, apply 2 to 3 diluted drops to the affected area. To prevent internal bacterial overgrowth, ingest 2 to 4 drops twice daily for up to 10 days.

4. Proves Effective Against MRSA and Staph Infection

Oregano is the oil of choice for acute MRSA and other staph infections. Add 3 drops of oregano oil to a capsule or to the food or beverage of your choice along with a carrier oil; take it twice daily for up to 10 days.

OREGANO USES

5. Fights Intestinal Worms and Parasites

Because oregano oil has anti-parasitic and anti-viral properties, it can be used internally to combat parasitic infections. Take oregano oil internally for up to 10 days.

6. Helps Removes Warts

One of the more common uses of oregano oil is its ability to safely diminish and possibly remove warts. When using oregano oil for removing warts, make sure to dilute it with another oil or mix it with clay.

7. Cleanses Mold From the Home

Oregano is effective at eradicating mold growth around your home. Add 5 to 7 drops to a homemade cleaning solution along with tea tree oil and lavender.

RESEARCH STUDIES

Twenty clinical strains of bacteria were tested on patients with different clinical conditions. Oregano oil was active against all tested strains. It proved to be an effective means for the prevention of antibiotic-resistant strain development.[20]

A 2014 study found that oregano oil has powerful anti-viral properties against non-enveloped murine norovirus, a human norovirus surrogate, in some cases inactivating the virus within an hour of exposure.[21]

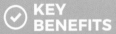

KEY BENEFITS

- Contains anti-bacterial and anti-fungal properties
- Helps prevent and treat viral infections
- Fights inflammation
- Helps relieve allergy symptoms
- Has shown promising anti-tumor properties
- Boosts the immune system
- Aids the respiratory system

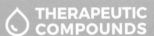

THERAPEUTIC COMPOUNDS

Carvacrol   Thymol

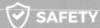

SAFETY

Avoid use during pregnancy—as oregano oil may cause embryotoxicity—or on infants and small children. It may cause skin irritation when used topically, so dilute it with a carrier oil and test on a small patch of skin first. If using internally, do not use for more than 10 days. After 10 days, take a break for one week.

PEPPERMINT

MENTHA PIPERITA

Peppermint is one of the oldest European herbs used for medicinal purposes, and historical accounts date its use to ancient Egyptian, Chinese and Japanese folk medicine. In ancient Greece, mint was used in funerary rites, together with rosemary and myrtle, and not simply to offset the smell of decay. In the Bible, mint is referenced along with anise and cumin to be given as a tithe to the Lord, demonstrating its value during that time.

A cross between a variety of wild mints, peppermint was more widely discovered in the 17th century. The essential oils are gathered by steam distillation of the fresh aerial parts of the flowering plant. Peppermint essential oil is used for its anti-nausea benefits and soothing effects on muscles, the colon and the gastric lining. It has a sharp, minty and intense aroma that serves as a stimulating and invigorating agent. Peppermint oil gives a cooling sensation and has a calming effect on the body, which can help relieve sore muscles and ease headaches when used topically. It also has anti-microbial properties, so it can help freshen bad breath and soothe digestive issues.

SUPER 7 RX

1. Helps Relieve Muscle Pain

Peppermint oil may help reduce pain and relax muscles. It is especially helpful in soothing an aching back, sore muscles and tension headaches. Dilute 2 to 4 drops and apply it topically to the area of concern.

2. Soothes Respiratory Conditions

Peppermint oil acts as an expectorant and may relieve some symptoms of a respiratory illness. Dilute 2 to 4 drops and apply it topically to your chest and the back of your neck. Alternatively, you can add 10 drops to boiling water, put a towel over your head and breathe in the aroma for 5 minutes.

3. Boosts Energy

Because peppermint is invigorating and stimulating, it can help fight chronic fatigue and improve concentration. Diffuse it, or apply it to your temples, wrists and the back of your neck. It can also be inhaled directly for a quick energy boost.

4. Helps Reduce Allergy Symptoms

Peppermint helps relax the muscles in the nasal passages and clear out mucus and pollen during allergy season. Diffuse 5 drops, inhale it directly from the bottle or dilute 2 to 3 drops and apply it topically to your forehead, neck and chest.

PEPPERMINT USES

5. Aids in Headache Relief

Peppermint oil may improve circulation, soothe the gut and relax tense muscles. It can also help clear your nasal passages when you're suffering from a sinus headache. Apply it to your forehead and temples for pain relief.

6. Eases Digestive Conditions

Peppermint oil helps to relax the muscles in the intestines and reduce bloating, gas and nausea. It may also serve as a natural remedy for irritable bowel syndrome. Diffuse it, apply it topically to your abdomen, or take 1 to 2 drops internally.

7. Freshens Breath and Fights Cavities

Peppermint oil has anti-microbial properties that will freshen breath and may kill bacteria that lead to cavities and gum disease. Add 1 drop to toothpaste or mouthwash, or place the oil under your tongue before drinking a glass of water.

RESEARCH STUDIES

A 2007 study used peppermint oil to treat irritable bowel syndrome. After four weeks, patients reported an average 50 percent reduction in symptoms, including abdominal bloating, abdominal discomfort, diarrhea, constipation and pain during elimination.[22]

A 1994 study found that a combination of peppermint and eucalyptus oil has significant effects on mechanisms associated with the pathophysiology of headaches.[23]

KEY BENEFITS

- Soothes digestive issues
- Freshens breath
- Helps relieve headaches
- Provides mental focus
- Promotes respiratory cleansing
- Boosts energy
- Eases tight muscles
- Helps relieve nausea and vomiting

THERAPEUTIC COMPOUNDS

Menthol   Menthone

SAFETY

Some medications may adversely interact with peppermint oil, so consult a physician with concerns about drug interactions.

ROSEMARY

ROSMARINUS OFFICINALIS

As a member of the mint family, rosemary has long been used as a powerful natural health booster. A tea made from rosemary leaves was once used to quiet nerves and strengthen memory, and the leaves are also used in perfumery and cooking. As early as 1584, rosemary was used as a symbol of remembrance on particular occasions such as funerals and weddings, or even as a decoration for brides. Shakespeare made reference to rosemary in *Hamlet* where Ophelia, decked with flowers, says to Laertes: "There's rosemary, that's for remembrance."

Rosemary's history extends further back than Shakespeare. The Ancient Egyptians, Romans and Greeks all considered it sacred, and it was widely used to cleanse the air and prevent sickness from spreading. It was used in folk medicine to improve memory, soothe digestive issues and relieve muscle aches and pains. More recently, it has been shown to boost nerve growth factor and support the healing of neurological tissue as well as boost brain function. Rosemary essential oil has a woody, evergreen-like scent and is steam-distilled from the leaves of the plant.

SUPER 7 RX

1. Increases Hair Growth

Rosemary essential oil stimulates hair growth and can help prevent baldness, slow graying and treat dandruff or dry scalp. Apply 3 to 5 drops to your scalp, rub it in and allow the oil to sit for 5 minutes before rinsing, or add 5 to 10 drops to shampoo or conditioner.

2. May Improve Memory

Studies show that rosemary oil improves cognitive performance, increases alertness and enhances overall quality of memory. Add it to a diffuser, or apply it topically under your nose or across your forehead.

3. Acts as a Natural Diabetes Remedy

Over time, incorporating rosemary oil into your daily routine can help to supplement and assist in the body's balance and regulation of hormones and blood sugar levels. Take 1 to 2 drops in a glass of water.

4. Helps Reduce Pain

Because of rosemary oil's anti-inflammatory properties, it has the power to reduce joint and muscle pain. Mix 2 drops of rosemary oil, 2 drops of peppermint oil and 1 teaspoon of coconut oil and rub it onto sore muscles and painful joints.

5. Promotes Liver Detox and Gallbladder Function

Using rosemary oil topically can enhance the performance of the bile-producing gallbladder and help to prevent toxin buildup in the body. Mix 3 drops of rosemary oil with ¼ teaspoon of coconut oil and rub it over your gallbladder area twice daily.

6. Aids in Detoxifying the Body

Rosemary oil boosts nutrient absorption and helps to reverse or prevent toxic overload. Take it internally, or apply 2 to 3 drops to your abdomen to detoxify your body.

7. Fights Respiratory Issues

Rosemary oil works as an expectorant—reducing mucus and relieving some of the symptoms of bronchitis, cold and other respiratory infections. Apply it topically to your chest, or diffuse it, to thin and expel mucus.

RESEARCH STUDIES

A 2012 study evaluated rosemary oil's effect on cognitive performance and mood. Twenty healthy volunteers performed tasks in a cubicle diffused with rosemary. Test results showed improved performance at higher concentrations of rosemary essential oil.[24]

Rosemary was found to be active against certain pathogenic bacteria and drug-resistant mutants of E. coli. Similarly, it was found to be highly active against pathogenic fungi and drug-resistant mutants of Candida albicans.[25]

KEY BENEFITS

· Relieves muscle aches and pains
· Contains anti-inflammatory properties
· Promotes hormone balance
· Soothes respiratory conditions
· Improves alertness
· Regenerates nerve tissue
· Thickens hair
· May improve memory

THERAPEUTIC COMPOUNDS

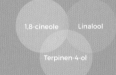

1,8-cineole   Linalool

Terpinen-4-ol

SAFETY

Use rosemary oil minimally during pregnancy. Do not use it if you have high blood pressure or if you've been diagnosed with epilepsy.

SPIKENARD

NARDOSTACHYS JATAMANSI

In ancient times, spikenard essential oil (also known as "nard") was regarded as one of the most precious oils. Many say that Solomon prophesied a thousand years earlier of Christ's victory over death using a reference to spikenard. Song of Solomon 1:12 says, "While the king sat at his table, my spikenard sent forth its fragrance." According to some scholars, the seated position of the King is symbolic of His finished work at Calvary's tree. He is inviting His bride (the church) to come and join Him at the marriage supper feast. The bride's fragrance emanates out of her spirit in worship and adoration for the King's provision.

Spikenard was also used in Greek and Roman healing and ceremonies, and it was even used in medieval cookery. Used in Ayurveda, it's great for both healing and a deep connection to spirit. For those suffering from anxiety, spikenard can soothe the nerves and quiet the mind. Spikenard oil is used to treat insomnia, stress, digestive problems and infections. The roots of the plant are steam-distilled to extract the essential oil, which has a heavy, sweet, woody and spicy aroma—said to resemble the smell of moss.

SUPER 7 RX

1. Displays Antibiotic Properties

When applied topically to wounds, spikenard can fight bacteria. Inside the body, spikenard helps treat bacterial infections in the kidneys, bladder and urethra. Apply 3 to 5 drops topically to the area of concern, or take 1 to 2 drops internally for infection and diffuse.

2. Can Reduce Inflammation

Spikenard oil relieves inflammation, which is at the root of many conditions and diseases such as asthma, arthritis, Crohn's disease, Alzheimer's disease, cancer, cardiovascular disease, diabetes, high blood pressure, high cholesterol and Parkinson's disease. Apply 3 to 5 drops topically twice daily, diffuse the oil or take 1 drop internally each day.

3. Helps Reduce Stress and Anxiety

Spikenard oil is relaxing and soothing for the skin and mind; it's often used as a sedative and calming agent. Diffuse spikenard oil or apply it topically.

4. Boosts the Immune System

Spikenard oil is an immune system booster because it calms the body, enabling it to function properly. To boost your immune system, diffuse spikenard or apply it topically to the soles of your feet or the back of your neck.

SPIKENARD USES

5. Promotes Hair Growth

Spikenard oil is known for promoting hair growth, helping to retain its natural color and slowing down the process of graying. Add 5 to 10 drops to a bottle of shampoo or conditioner, or combine 5 drops of spikenard oil with 1 teaspoon of coconut oil and massage the mixture into your scalp; let it sit for 5 minutes before rinsing.

6. Treats Insomnia

Spikenard's sedative and relaxing properties can be helpful to those with insomnia or sleep deprivation. Diffuse or apply 2 to 3 drops topically to your temples and the back of your neck.

7. Helps with Constipation

Spikenard oil is a natural laxative, and it stimulates the digestive system, helping to naturally relieve constipation. Apply spikenard oil onto your stomach and the soles of your feet.

RESEARCH STUDIES

A 2008 study done on mice found that spikenard extract had sedative and calming benefits.[26]

Study results indicate that spikenard oil shows a positive response in hair growth promotion activity, showing that spikenard may work as a hair loss remedy.[27]

KEY BENEFITS
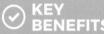

- May reduce inflammation
- Fights bacteria and fungi
- Can relax the body and mind
- Boosts the immune system
- Helps protect the uterus and ovaries
- May improve insomnia
- Boosts skin and hair health

THERAPEUTIC COMPOUNDS
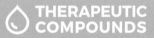

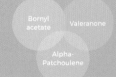

Bornyl acetate

Valeranone

Alpha-Patchoulene

SAFETY
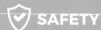

Do not use during pregnancy since spikenard oil can stimulate the uterus.

CARRIER OILS

Carrier oils are used to dilute essential oils when they are being used topically; they help to *carry* the essential oils into the skin. Many lotions and skin care products are made with carrier oils, which are vegetable oils derived from the fatty portion of the plant, like the nuts, kernels or seeds. Unlike essential oils, carrier oils do not evaporate easily and do not give off strong aromas. Unfortunately, carrier oils often have a defined shelf life and will become rancid over time.

Each carrier oil offers a different combination of nourishing properties, benefits and characteristics. Some are more aromatic than others, and the color and shelf life will differ as well. The following pages will provide you with some of the most widely used carrier oils that can be combined with essential oils in aromatherapy.

Almond

Almond oil presents a variety of health benefits: It addresses bad cholesterol, helps prevent inflammation, hydrates dry skin and supports cardiovascular health. This oil has even been presented as an alternative, renewable biofuel source. When used topically, it is known for its ability to soften and soothe inflamed skin. It absorbs into the skin fairly quickly, leaving a slight hint of oil.

Apricot Kernel

The kernels of the apricot fruit are cold-pressed to extract the beneficial oils. This oil works great as a massage oil because it is very light and soothing to the skin. In Traditional Chinese Medicine, apricot kernel oil is used to treat tumors and ulcers. It has also been used to relieve digestive issues and boost skin health.

Arnica

Arnica oil has been used for medicinal purposes since the 1500s. It contains helenalin, a potent anti-inflammatory agent, which is why arnica oil is commonly used on the skin in the form of an oil, cream, ointment, liniment or salve. This carrier oil needs to be diluted before topical use. When purchased from a store, arnica oil should already be diluted and ready for use, but make sure to read the label carefully. When applied to the skin, it helps to reduce pain caused by inflammation, while also treating bruises, aches, sprains and even arthritis flare-ups.

Argan

For generations, natives of the Argan Forest in Morocco have pressed the argan nut to extract this precious oil to use as a dietary supplement for wound healing and rash relief, and to nourish skin and hair. Argan oil is rich in vitamins A and E; it is also packed with antioxidants, omega-6 fatty acids and linoleic acid. When it is applied topically, it eases inflammation, moisturizes skin and boosts cell production.

Avocado

Avocado oil has actually received prescription drug status in France because of its proven ability to counter the negative effects of arthritis. This oil is produced from the fruit of the avocado tree. Because it is extracted from the fleshy pulp of the fruit, it is one of the few edible oils not derived from a seed. The pulp produces oil full of healthy fats, including oleic acid and essential fatty acids. Avocado oil can be used topically to hydrate dry hair and improve its texture, as well as improve skin health. It also reduces inflammation and boosts nutrient absorption.

Coconut

The coconut tree is considered the "tree of life" in much of Southeast Asia, India, the Philippines and other tropical locations. Today, there are over 1,500 articles demonstrating the health benefits of coconut oil. The uses are numerous thanks to its natural healing properties and tremendous use as a product for natural beauty treatments and so much more.

Evening Primrose

Primrose is a wild flower that grows in eastern and central North America. The seeds of the flower are cold-pressed for the extraction of their oil, which is high in essential fatty acids. Evening primrose oil has a range of therapeutic properties; it is known to help reduce the pain associated with PMS and relieve skin irritations and conditions. The oil could also be used as an anti-inflammatory agent, and it is commonly used to relieve problems with autoimmune diseases.

Hemp

Hemp seed is an all-natural way to jumpstart better skin with a wave of incredible vitamins. Hemp seed oil does not contain THC (tetrahydrocannabinol) or the other psychoactive constituents that are present in the dried leaves of Cannabis sativa. With generous amounts of omega fatty acids and proteins, this oil wonderfully reinvigorates the skin as it helps to clear away acne and eczema. Extremely emollient and absorbent, hemp seed oil is packed with vitamins A, B1, B2, B3, B6, C, D and E. It also has abundant levels of anti-inflammatory and antioxidant properties. Hemp seed oil also reduces toxins while alleviating sore muscles and joints.

Jojoba

Jojoba oil (pronounced ho-ho-ba) is the liquid that comes from the seed of the Simmondsia chinensis plant. It is labeled as an oil, but is actually a liquid plant wax that has been used in folk medicine for a number of ailments. Because jojoba is an emollient, it soothes the skin and unclogs hair follicles. It can be combined with essential oils such as lavender or peppermint to boost skin and hair health.

Olive

Olive trees have been around for many thousands of years. With a long history dating back to ancient civilizations, olive oil is even considered to be one of the most important Bible foods. High-quality olive oil has well-researched anti-inflammatory compounds and antioxidants. It is made from the fruit of the olive tree, which is naturally high in healthy fatty acids. When used topically, olive oil reduces oxidative damage and works as an anti-microbial agent. It should be used in small amounts, as the olive fragrance could overpower the aroma of essential oils when used in high doses.

Pomegranate

Pomegranate seed oil is considered one of the Bible's powerful foods because of its powerful anti-aging benefits. The dark red color in pomegranate seed oil comes from the bioflavonoids, which protect the skin from sun damage. It has a natural sun protection factor (SPF) and can be used as a sunblock and sunscreen.

Rosehip

Rosehip oil is harvested from the seeds of rose bushes predominately grown in Chile. It contains powerful antioxidants, vitamins and essential fatty acids—making it an effective carrier oil for hydrating the skin, relieving itchiness and minimizing the appearances of dark spots, scars and fine lines. Rosehip absorbs easily, and it is non-greasy and light when applied topically.

Sea Buckthorn

Sea buckthorn berries and seeds are cold-pressed and CO_2 extracted for their oils, which are rich in essential fatty acids and contain vitamins, minerals and nutritive compounds. Sea buckthorn oil is used on the skin to reduce the signs of aging. Because of its intense color that can stain skin when used in high doses, a 1:3 dilution is recommended.

Shea Butter

Shea butter is not a carrier oil, but its natural, beneficial properties make it a lipid suitable for aromatherapy work. It is highly moisturizing, has a smooth, creamy texture and can be included in massage blends, lotions, creams and other natural skin care products. Shea butter can become gritty if not melted and then cooled properly. Once it has cooled, it does not need to be kept in the refrigerator.

As you continue growing your collection of essential oils, experiment with different carrier oils; they have so many uses as both carriers and in DIY recipes. Find the ones that work best for you to get the most out of your essential oils' therapeutic qualities.

What About Mineral Oil?

Mineral oil and petroleum jelly are byproducts of petroleum production. They are not of natural, botanical origin and are not used within the scope of holistic therapy. Mineral oil is used in baby oils and many commercially available moisturizers because it is an inexpensive oil to manufacture. It can, however, clog pores, prevent the skin from breathing naturally, prevent essential oil absorption, prevent toxins from leaving the body through the natural process of sweating and may even block vitamins from properly being utilized.

RECIPES

We believe essential oils have the power to change the way you feel. While they are not cure-alls, the use of essential oils through aromatherapy, topical application and internal consumption has a variety of health benefits, providing you with non-invasive home remedies for a multitude of conditions. Even better, they can be used safely in combination with many other therapies.

Some traditional hospitals are catching on to the benefits of essential oils and are using them to aid patients who are being treated for conditions such as anxiety, depression and infections. A 2009 study found that pre-operative patients who received aromatherapy with lavandin oil were significantly less anxious about their surgery than those in the control group. Other oils such as sandalwood, neroli oil and lavender oil have also been used in traditional medicine to help patients better manage anxiety. [28]

Additionally, essential oils have been shown to help patients better manage pain. A 2007 study in the *Journal of Alternative and Complementary Medicine* found that women who used aromatherapy during labor reported less pain overall and were able to use fewer pain medications.[29]

Essential oils can also have anti-bacterial and anti-fungal benefits. When key oils are massaged into the skin, they can promote healing and fight harmful bacteria. Others may help boost the immune system, reduce symptoms of insomnia and aid with digestion.

For each oil, we recommend referring to its single oil page in Part II for recommended applications and safety guidelines.

If you are taking any prescription medications, please consult with your healthcare practitioner before use.

We hope you will use this section often as a reference guide in your quest for better health and a cleaner lifestyle that most closely resembles the way God intended for us to nourish our bodies inside and out.

The power of essential oils rests in their chemical compounds—and in this section, we have detailed the most common conditions from which Americans suffer. For each, we provide you with:

Background: A brief summary of the condition.
Essential Oils: The most effective essential oils for that condition.
Research: Documented research and clinical studies for key uses.
Home Remedy: A DIY remedy to help improve symptoms and promote natural healing.
Suggested Supplements: Two to three recommended supplements to help round out a wellness protocol.

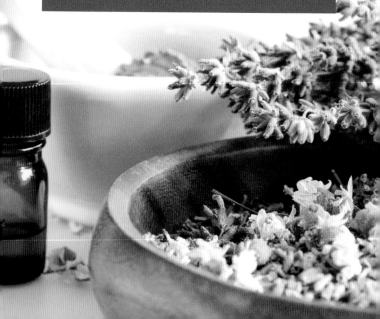

ALLERGIES

BACKGROUND

Today, 40 to 60 million Americans are affected by allergies—and the numbers continue to rise, especially in children. Allergies can cause a blocked and runny nose, sneezing, watery eyes, headaches and an impaired sense of smell. For some people, allergies can be life threatening, leading to acute inflammation and shortness of breath. People who suffer from allergies are often told to avoid triggers, but that is nearly impossible when the seasons are changing and our immune systems are impaired by improper diets and environmental toxins. Thankfully, key essential oils serve as a natural and safe way to address the symptoms of allergies and boost our immune systems.

Essential Oils

Eucalyptus. Aids in clearing the lungs and sinuses.

Peppermint. Unclogs sinuses and soothes scratchy throats.

Ginger. Contains anti-inflammatory properties that may improve symptoms of allergies.

Lemon. Supports lymphatic drainage and rids the body of impurities.

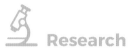

Research

A survey from NYU Medical School discovered that using eucalyptus helped deal with sinusitis. Patients experienced faster improvement whenever supplementing along with eucalyptus oil for allergies and sinus issues.[30]

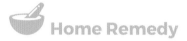

Home Remedy

Vapor Rub. Pour ¼ cup of olive oil, ½ cup of coconut oil and ¼ cup of grated beeswax into a glass jar. Place a saucepan with 2 inches of water over medium-low heat. Put the jar in the saucepan and allow the oils to melt. Allow it to cool slightly before adding 20 drops each of peppermint and eucalyptus. Pour the mixture into a metal tin and cool before use.

Suggested Supplements

> **Stinging Nettle.** A powerful herb with antihistamine properties.

> **Quercetin.** Shown to reduce symptoms of hay fever and seasonal allergies.

> **Spirulina.** Proven to significantly improve allergy symptoms, including nasal discharge, sneezing, nasal congestion and itching.[31]

ANXIETY

BACKGROUND

In today's fast-paced, high-pressure society, it's almost impossible not to feel anxious at some point in life. That is why an estimated 40 million American adults are affected by anxiety. For a person with an anxiety disorder, the anxiety does not go away and can get worse over time. These feelings can interfere with daily activities involving his or her job, schoolwork and relationships. Constant anxiety can lead to high blood pressure, insomnia, digestive problems and panic attacks. Some causes include stress, thyroid problems and hormone imbalance, as well as excessive alcohol, caffeine or sugar intake.

Essential Oils

Lavender. Aids neurological issues such as anxiety, migraines and depression.

Roman Chamomile. May ease feelings of paranoia and aggression.

Vetiver. Used for relaxation; helps to alleviate anxiety, insomnia and depression.

Frankincense. Shown to help reduce heart rate and high blood pressure.

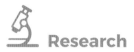

Research

A recent study found that supplementing with lavender essential oil alleviated anxiety, sleep disturbance and depression in participants; lavender oil treatment had no adverse side effects.[32]

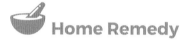

Home Remedy

Healing Bath Salts. Combine 3 cups of Epsom salt and 1 cup of baking soda. At bath time, add 1 cup of the dry ingredients and 20 to 30 drops of lavender to warm bath water. Soak for 20 to 30 minutes.

Suggested Supplements

▶ **Ashwagandha.** An adaptogenic herb; shown to improve anxiety symptoms by reducing the effects of stress on the body.[33]

▶ **Magnesium.** Known as the "relaxation mineral;" reduces tension and calms the nervous system. Take 500 milligrams daily or use magnesium oil topically.

ARTHRITIS

BACKGROUND

It is estimated that more than 52 million people in the U.S. suffer from arthritis symptoms. Arthritis can be defined as inflammation of one or more joints; the types of arthritis range from those related to wear and tear of cartilage (such as osteoarthritis) to those associated with inflammation resulting from an overactive immune system (such as rheumatoid arthritis). Symptoms vary greatly in intensity and include pain and limited function of joints. Essential oils may not only relieve pain but also improve your mood and overall health at the same time.

Essential Oils

Wintergreen. Acts as a natural analgesic to relieve pain and swelling.

Peppermint. Natural analgesic and muscle relaxant; helps soothe joint discomfort.

Frankincense and Turmeric. Reduce inflammation; help improve circulation.

Ginger. Reduces prostaglandins in the body (compounds associated with pain).[34]

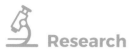

Research

A 2013 study concluded that ginger oil possesses antioxidant activity as well as significant anti-inflammatory and pain-reducing properties.[35]

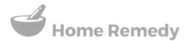

Home Remedy

Detoxifying Arthritis Bath. Run a warm-water bath and add 2 cups of Epsom salt, plus 20 drops of lavender with 20 drops of peppermint and soak for as long as desired. For added benefit, diffuse frankincense while you are soaking.

Suggested Supplements

▶ **Fish Oil.** An 18-month study showed that taking fish oil "exhibited significant reductions" in arthritis activity.[36] Take 1,000 milligrams of high-quality fish oil daily.

▶ **Turmeric.** A powerful anti-inflammatory herb; supplement with 1,000 milligrams per day.

BUG BITES

BACKGROUND

Many insects and spiders bite or sting, and while the bites of common bugs such as mosquitoes, mites and fleas are itchy and uncomfortable, they're usually harmless. But some bites and stings, such as those from fire ants, wasps, hornets and bees, may cause intense pain or even an allergic reaction. Others, such as poisonous spider bites, may require immediate emergency medical care. Certain oils have the power to soothe the skin and fight possible infections from insects. Essential oils can also ward off bugs; use them to make a homemade bug spray—they will help to fight bacteria and nourish the skin, too.

Essential Oils

  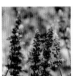

Citronella. Acts as an all-natural bug repellant.

Lemongrass. Repels bugs such as mosquitoes because of its high citral and geraniol content.

Lavender. Feels soothing when applied directly to the skin; can help speed up the healing process.

Holy Basil. Has wound healing abilities, largely due to the presence of eugenol.[37]

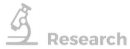

Research

A 2016 study tested the effects of the oils of certain plants against mosquito bites. The oils of citrus leaves, citrus fruit peel and Alpinia galanga (rhizome) were used to create a lotion and compared against commercial repellants. The essential oil-based lotions revealed an impressive 90 percent protection against mosquito bites for four hours.[38]

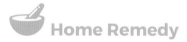

Home Remedy

Bug Spray. Mix ½ cup of witch hazel, ½ cup of apple cider vinegar and 40 drops of essential oils (a mix of citronella, eucalyptus, lemongrass and tea tree) in a spray bottle. Spray your body, avoiding your eyes and mouth.

Suggested Supplements

▶ **Witch Hazel.** Can help reduce the pain, annoying itching and swelling associated with bug bites; may speed up the healing process.

▶ **Colloidal Silver + Oatmeal Bath.** Soothes the itching caused by mosquito bites; reduces swelling from bites.

COMMON COLD

BACKGROUND

According to estimates, adults and children in the U.S. get 1 billion colds each year. There are over 200 viruses that can cause a cold. Cold viruses take up residence in the lining of the nose and grow, eventually attempting to infect the body. If the body is weak or unable to resist the germs, it will get sick. Despite what some people think, there's no evidence that cold weather, large tonsils or other such wives' tales can make you "catch" a cold.[39] Evidence does suggest that stress and allergies can increase your chances of getting a cold. Colds generally last from about two days to two weeks. Some common symptoms of a cold include runny or stuffy nose, low-grade fever, sore throat, cough and body aches.

Essential Oils

Thyme. Helps drain congestion; proven to fight infections and rid the body of toxins.[40]

Lemon. Can support lymphatic drainage and help to overcome a cold quickly.

Ginger. Relieves discomfort caused by congestion and infections.

Eucalyptus & Peppermint. Work as expectorants and help cleanse the body.

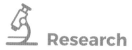

Research

According to a 2002 study, d-limonene (a primary compound found in lemon oil) directly activates the immune response of alveolar phagocytes. Phagocytes are cells that protect the body by ingesting harmful foreign particles, bacteria and dead or dying cells.[41]

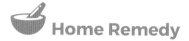

Home Remedy

Steam Bath. Make a steam bath by mixing 10 drops each of eucalyptus oil and peppermint oil, placing a towel over your head and inhaling deeply for 5 to 10 minutes.

Suggested Supplements

▶ **Echinacea and Elderberry.** Act as anti-inflammatories, helping reduce symptoms of cold and flu.

▶ **Garlic.** Some studies suggest supplementing with garlic will lead to fewer colds and faster recovery.[42]

DEPRESSION

BACKGROUND

Depression is a common but serious mood disorder caused by changes in brain chemistry. It affects approximately 14.8 million American adults. Depression causes severe symptoms that affect how you feel, think and handle daily activities. Symptoms include fatigue, sadness, low sex drive, lack of appetite, feelings of helplessness and disinterest in common activities. Research indicates that other factors contribute to the onset of depression, including genetics, changes in hormone levels, certain medical conditions, stress, grief or difficult life circumstances. Antidepressant medications have serious side effects that can include suicidal thoughts, weight gain and personality changes; what's worse, studies have shown that antidepressants fail to cure the symptoms of major depression in half of all treated patients.

Essential Oils

Bergamot. Can create feelings of joy and energy by improving circulation of the blood.[43]

Ylang Ylang. Acts as a mild sedative and can lower stress responses.

Lavender. Known to aid neurological conditions, including depression and anxiety.

Roman Chamomile. Inhaling it may help lessen anxiety and general depression.

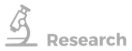 **Research**

A 2012 study took 28 high-risk postpartum women and found that after a four-week treatment plan of lavender aromatherapy, they had a significant reduction of postnatal depression and reduced anxiety disorder.[44]

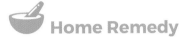 **Home Remedy**

Invigorating Inhalation. Rub 1 drop each of bergamot oil, lavender oil and ylang ylang oil into your hands and cup your mouth and nose. Breathe in the oil slowly. Also try rubbing the oils on your feet and stomach.

Suggested Supplements

▶ **Fish Oil.** High in EPA, which is critical for neurotransmitter function—an important component in emotional and physiological brain balance.

▶ **Vitamin D3.** Helps improve seasonal affective disorder (may manifest as depression).

HEADACHES

Headaches are an extremely common ailment that affects millions of people across the globe. It has been estimated that up to three-quarters of adults have had a headache at least once within the last year. A headache is a good indicator that the body is missing something—it may be the result of dehydration, nutrient deficiency or a food sensitivity that is causing this built-up tension. A multitude of headache triggers exist, including stress, fatigue, allergies, eyestrain, poor posture, alcohol or drugs, low blood sugar, hormones, constipation and nutritional deficiencies. The most severe form of a headache is known as a migraine, which can cause vision disturbance and vomiting.

Essential Oils

Peppermint. Improves circulation and reduces pain.[45]

Lavender. Reduces muscle tension; used as a mood stabilizer, sedative and effective migraine remedy.

Eucalyptus. Opens nasal airways; eliminates sinus pressure that can lead to headaches.

Rosemary. Stimulating, anti-inflammatory and analgesic.

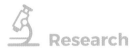

Research

A 2012 study measured the results of inhaling lavender oil for 15 minutes. The 47 participants were asked to record the effects every half hour, for two hours. Out of 129 headache attacks, 92 responded positively to the lavender oil remedy.[46]

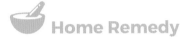

Home Remedy

Headache Ease. Rub a mixture of peppermint oil, lavender oil and a carrier oil on your temples, chest and the back of your neck. Before washing your hands after application, cup your hands and breathe in deeply for several minutes.

Suggested Supplements

▶ **Magnesium.** Migraine sufferers have lower levels of magnesium both during and between attacks compared with healthy individuals.[47]

▶ **Feverfew.** Reduces the frequency of migraine headaches and headache symptoms, including pain, nausea, vomiting and sensitivity to light and noise.[48]

HEARTBURN

BACKGROUND

Heartburn is a form of indigestion caused by acid regurgitation into the esophagus. Often considered a symptom of acid reflux, the most common times to experience heartburn occur in the evening after a heavy meal, during movement such as bending or lifting or when lying down. Symptoms include burning or pain in the chest, stomachaches after eating, a bitter taste in the mouth, belching and nausea. Roughly 20 percent of American adults endure painful heartburn on a weekly basis—and yet many are unaware of simple and natural remedies that work quickly to correct the underlying digestive problem, as diet and lifestyle habits are the biggest contributors to heartburn.

Essential Oils

Ginger. Blocks the production of acid and helps prevent ulcers.

Peppermint. Relaxes the muscles, allowing painful digestive gas to pass.[49]

Fennel. Balances the pH level within the body, especially within the stomach.

Lemon. Helps temporarily excrete digestive acids.

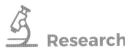 **Research**

A 2015 study reported that ginger essential oil treatment inhibited ulcers in laboratory animals by 85 percent, suggesting the promising gastro-protective activity of ginger.[50]

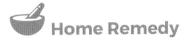 **Home Remedy**

Heartburn Quick Fix. Add 1 drop each of peppermint and lemon essential oils to a tablespoon of apple cider vinegar plus a spoonful of honey for a soothing way to combat digestive issues.

Suggested Supplements

▶ **Raw Apple Cider Vinegar.** Naturally acidic; lowers the pH in your stomach. Take 1 tablespoon before meals.

▶ **HCL with Pepsin.** Increases the level of acid in the stomach necessary for proper digestion. (Only take with meals that contain protein; do NOT use if you take corticosteroids or anti-inflammatory medications such as NSAIDs.)

▶ **Digestive Enzymes.** Help break down hard-to-digest starches and proteins.

IMMUNE DEFENSE

BACKGROUND

The immune system is a network of cells, tissues and organs that work together to protect the body from infection. Your immune system does a remarkable job of defending against disease-causing microorganisms, but it isn't perfect—some germs invade successfully and make you sick. However, it is possible to intervene in this process and make your immune system stronger. Some essential oils have the power to target invading microbes, infected cells and even tumors—protecting the body from disease and other health conditions.

Essential Oils

Frankincense. Has superior immune-boosting ability; multiplies white blood cells.[51]

Thyme. Has anti-viral and immune-boosting compounds that protect the body.

Orange. Contains limonene, which is a powerful defender against oxidative stress.

Myrrh. Contains anti-inflammatory properties.

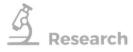

Research

In a clinical study on chickens, thyme essential oil was found to reduce the incidence of disease.[52]

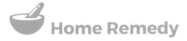

Home Remedy

Immune-Boosting Juice. Extract the juice of 1 bell pepper, 1 head/stem of broccoli and 1 cucumber. Mix the juice in a blender with 1 to 2 drops of lemon oil or orange oil, 1 to 2 drops of ginger oil and 1 tablespoon of apple cider vinegar.

Suggested Supplements

▶ **Probiotics.** Line your digestive tract and support your body's ability to absorb nutrients and fight infection.

▶ **Bone Broth Protein Powder.** Contains type 2 collagen, which helps repair gut lining and improves immunity.

INFECTION

An infection is the invasion of body tissues by disease-causing agents. These agents are able to multiply, cause a reaction in bodily tissues and produce toxins within the body. An infection can lead to countless symptoms, from a sore throat and fever to far more serious and sometimes fatal complications. Worldwide, infectious diseases are the leading cause of death of children and adolescents, and one of the leading causes in adults. Infections are caused by germs such as viruses, bacteria, parasites and fungi. Many of the constituents in essential oils have been proven to fight these germs and help you recover from or possibly evade infection.

Essential Oils

   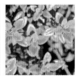

Oregano. Has proven and powerful antibiotic capabilities.[53]

Cedarwood. Defends the body against toxins; fights off bacteria in the body.

Tea Tree & Manuka. Destroys parasites and fungi.

Thyme. An antiseptic; controls infections on the skin and within the body; antibacterial.[54]

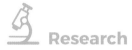

Research

A study conducted at the Department of Oral Medicine and Radiology found that cedarwood is effective in controlling both bacteria and yeasts responsible for oral infections.[55]

Home Remedy

Infection-Fighting Lotion. Mix 1 to 2 drops each of tea tree, cedarwood, manuka and thyme oils into a squirt of natural lotion and apply it to areas of infection or to your lymph nodes to fight internal infection. Additionally, take oregano oil internally for up to two weeks.

Suggested Supplements

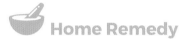

▶ **Elderberry.** Fights infections, including influenza, herpes, viral infections and bacterial infections.

▶ **Echinacea.** Evidence suggests that phytochemicals in echinacea have the capacity to reduce viral infections.[56]

MUSCLE ACHES

BACKGROUND

A muscle cramp is an involuntarily and forcibly contracted muscle that does not relax. Most people experience a muscle cramp at some time in their life. There is a variety of types and causes of muscle cramps. One of the most common causes of muscle cramps is dehydration, but other causes include increased physical activity or a lack of activity, stress, nutritional deficiencies and hormonal changes. The body may not be getting enough electrolytes, such as potassium or magnesium. Some other medical explanations include fibromyalgia, statin drugs, flu symptoms, hormonal changes and Lyme disease. Essential oils such as peppermint and cypress are ideal home remedies for muscle aches and pains.

Essential Oils

Peppermint and Wintergreen. Effective natural pain relievers and muscle relaxants.

Cypress. A sedative with a calming and relaxing effect on the body.

Marjoram and Lemongrass. May reduce muscle spasms and muscle pain.

Lavender. Indicated for muscular spasms, cramps, sprains and rheumatism.[57]

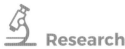

Research

A study shows that peppermint oil applied topically has pain relief benefits associated with fibromyalgia and myofascial pain syndrome. The study found that peppermint, eucalyptus, menthol, capsaicin and other herbal preparations may be helpful.[58]

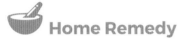

Home Remedy

Muscle Compress. Put 3 drops of peppermint oil, 3 drops of cypress oil and 1 teaspoon of coconut oil on the area of concern, and then cover it with a hot compress for 3 to 5 minutes.

Suggested Supplements

▶ **Magnesium.** Can help with muscle relaxation. Take 250 milligrams twice daily.

▶ **Bone Broth Protein Powder.** Supports healthy joints and muscles and promotes tissue repair.

NAUSEA

BACKGROUND

Almost everyone at some point in life has experienced symptoms of nausea, that sick feeling in your stomach that often comes just before vomiting. There are many causes of nausea, but some of the most common include pregnancy, food poisoning, motion sickness, flu symptoms, gallbladder distress, medications, migraine headaches and emotional stress. Morning sickness is nausea and/or vomiting that occurs during pregnancy. The timing of the nausea or vomiting can sometimes indicate the cause. For example, when it appears shortly after a meal, nausea or vomiting may be caused by food poisoning, gastritis (inflammation of the stomach lining) or an ulcer. If nausea leads to severe vomiting, dehydration becomes a concern. The next time your stomach is uneasy, use essential oils for natural relief.

Essential Oils

Peppermint. Can reduce nausea, as well as bloating and gas.

Ginger. Known to reduce nausea and upset stomach.[59]

Basil. An anti-spasmodic that can lessen cramps associated with motion sickness.[60]

Lavender. Works as a mild sedative; helps to relax the body during times of stress.

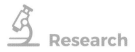

Research

A medical study found that peppermint oil use reduced chemotherapy-induced nausea better than standard medical treatments.[61]

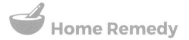

Home Remedy

Nausea Ease. Rub peppermint, ginger and lavender oils behind your ears or on your stomach, or take it internally to help relieve nausea.

Suggested Supplements

▶ **Vitamin B6.** Helps reduce nausea. Take 25 milligrams, three times daily.

▶ **Digestive Enzymes.** Help the body digest macronutrients and can reduce symptoms of nausea when consumed consistently. Take 1 to 3 capsules daily with meals.

WEIGHT GAIN/ OBESITY

BACKGROUND

"Overweight" and "obesity" are both labels for ranges of weight that are greater than what is generally considered healthy for a given height. The terms also identify ranges of weight that have been shown to increase the likelihood of certain diseases and other health problems. More than 35 percent of U.S. adults are obese, and more than 34 percent are overweight for a combined total of a whopping 69 percent.[62] An adult who has a BMI between 25 and 29.9 is considered overweight. An adult who has a BMI of 30 or higher is considered obese. Excess weight is often caused by an overconsumption of calories and physical inactivity. Some other causes may include hormonal imbalances, stress, medical conditions, genetics, toxins or certain medications. The good news is there are steps to treat weight gain and obesity naturally, which include eating a healthy diet, doing weekly exercise and using natural supplements.

Essential Oils

Cinnamon. Contains cinnamaldehyde, which promotes healthy blood sugar.

Grapefruit. May reduce cravings for sweets and improve metabolism.

Ginger. Helps reduce systemic inflammation and improve digestion.

Black Pepper. Naturally warms the body; stimulates metabolism.[63]

Research

In a study, the scent of grapefruit oil stimulated loss of body fat, strengthened adrenal function and reduced appetite in laboratory animals. Researchers concluded grapefruit oil has tremendous potential as a weight loss aid.[64]

Home Remedy

Weight Loss Boost. Add 1 to 3 drops of grapefruit oil to a glass of water three times daily, or add a blend of cinnamon, grapefruit, ginger and black pepper to a diffuser and take in deep breaths for two minutes, one to three times daily.

Suggested Supplements

▶ **Bone Broth Protein Powder.** High in easy-to-digest protein, which may support healthy blood sugar and metabolism.

▶ **Probiotics.** Studies have shown improved weight loss with probiotic use; helps clear excess yeast, which may contribute to food cravings.

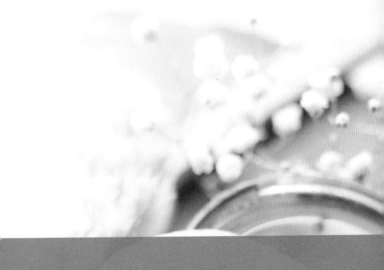

PERSONAL CARE

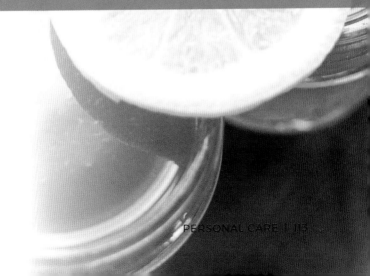

ANTI-AGING SERUM

Time: 2 minutes   Serves: 15 uses

INGREDIENTS

- ½ tablespoon jojoba oil
- ½ tablespoon evening primrose oil
- ½ tablespoon pomegranate oil
- 20 drops lavender essential oil or frankincense essential oil
- 15 drops vitamin E oil
- 10 drops carrot seed essential oil

DIRECTIONS

1. In a small bowl, mix all ingredients.
2. Transfer the serum into a dark glass bottle. Use it every morning and night on your face, neck and chest.

DEODORANT

Time: 5 minutes   Serves: 30-90 uses

INGREDIENTS

- ¼ cup baking soda
- ¼ cup coconut oil
- ¼ cup grated beeswax
- ¼ cup shea butter
- 3 tablespoons arrowroot powder
- 40 drops essential oils of your choice*

*Note: Recommended female oils scents—ylang ylang, jasmine, lavender and lemon; recommended male oils scents—sandalwood, bergamot, black pepper and cypress.

DIRECTIONS

1. Over a double broiler, melt the coconut or arnica oil and beeswax together. Stir gently until completely melted.
2. Add in the remaining ingredients and stir again.
3. Once mixed, quickly poor the mixture into an empty deodorant container.
4. Keep the container upright and allow the mixture to cool and harden before use.

HAND SANITIZER

Time: 2 minutes   Serves: 30 uses

INGREDIENTS

- 3 tablespoons aloe vera gel
- 1 tablespoon filtered water
- 5 drops tea tree essential oil
- 1 teaspoon vitamin E

DIRECTIONS

1. In a small bowl, add all ingredients and mix.
2. Transfer the mixture into a BPA-free plastic squeeze bottle and use as needed.

MUSCLE RUB

Time: 30 minutes   Serves: 30 uses

INGREDIENTS

- ½ cup coconut oil or arnica oil
- ¼ cup grated beeswax
- 2 teaspoons cayenne powder
- 15 drops ginger essential oil
- 15 drops peppermint essential oil
- 15 drops helichrysum essential oil

DIRECTIONS

1. In a small saucepan, add 2 inches of water. Place over medium-low heat.
2. In a glass jar, add the coconut oil and beeswax. Place the jar in the saucepan and stir, allowing the mixture to melt. Add the cayenne and ginger.
3. Once combined, allow the mixture to cool slightly. Mix in the essential oils.
4. Pour the mixture into metal tins or glass storage containers. Allow it to set.

SLEEP SERUM

Time: 2 minutes   Serves: 30-60 uses

INGREDIENTS

2 drops Roman chamomile essential oil

2 drops lavender essential oil

2 drops ylang ylang essential oil

Fractionated coconut oil, as needed

DIRECTIONS

1. In a small roll-on glass bottle, combine the essential oils.

2. Top off the mixture with the fractionated coconut oil.

3. Roll the mixture onto your neck at night right before going to sleep.

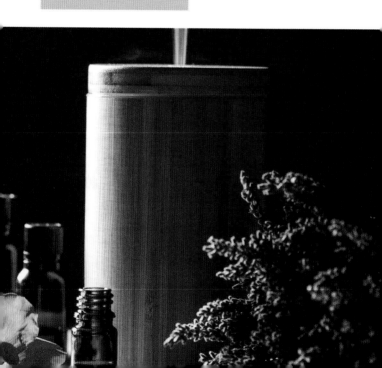

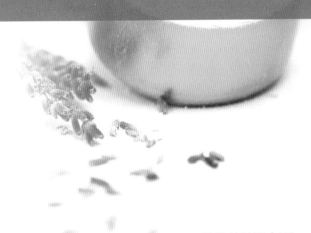

FOR THE HOME

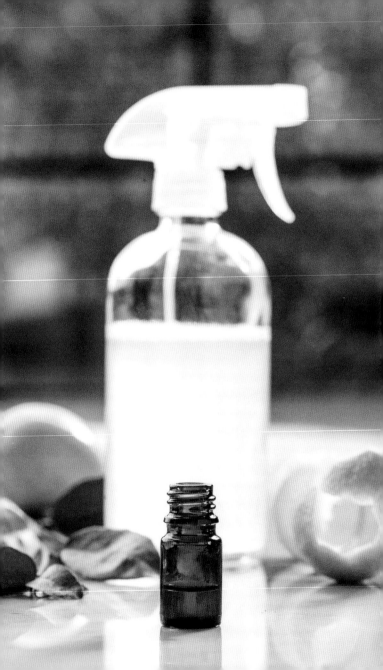

HOUSEHOLD CLEANER

Time: 2 minutes   Serves: 30-60 uses

INGREDIENTS

- 8 ounces water
- 4 ounces distilled white vinegar
- 15 drops melaleuca essential oil
- 15 drops lemon essential oil

DIRECTIONS

1. In a glass spray bottle, mix all ingredients.
2. Swirl or shake the bottle before each spray.

LAUNDRY SOAP

Time: 5 minutes   Serves: 12-15 uses

INGREDIENTS

- 1 bar Castile soap, grated
- 2 cups borax
- 2 cups washing soda
- 1 cup baking soda
- 15 drops lavender essential oil
- 15 drops peppermint essential oil

DIRECTIONS

1. In an airtight container, combine all ingredients and store.
2. Use ¼ cup per large load of laundry (adjust accordingly for smaller loads).

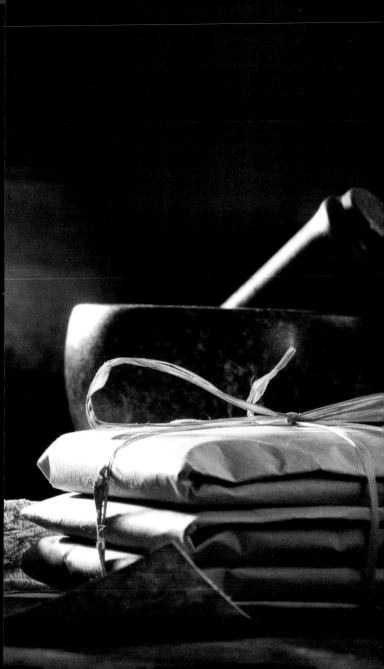

ENDNOTES

1   Chung, J.W., Kim, J.J., Kim, S.J. (2011, October). Antioxidative effects of cinnamomi cortex: A potential role of iNOS and COX-II. *Pharmacogn Mag.* Retrieved from http://www.ncbi.nlm.nih.gov/pmc/articles/PMC3261065/

2   Al-Mariri, A., Saour, G., Hamou, R. (2012, June). In Vitro Antibacterial Effects of Five Volatile Oil Extracts Against Intramacrophage Brucella Abortus 544. *Iran J Med Sci.* Retrieved from http://www.ncbi.nlm.nih.gov/pmc/articles/PMC3470071/

3   Burns, E., Blamey, C., Ersser. S.J., Lloyd, A.J., Barnetson, L. (2000, February). The use of aromatherapy in intrapartum midwifery practice an observational study. *Complement Ther Nurs Midwifery.* Retrieved from http://www.ncbi.nlm.nih.gov/pubmed/11033651

4   Sienkiewicz, M., Głowacka, A., Poznańska-Kurowska, K., Kaszuba, A., Urbaniak, A., Kowalczyk, E. (2015, February 3). The effect of clary sage oil on staphylococci responsible for wound infections. *Postepy Dermatol Alergol.* Retrieved from http://www.ncbi.nlm.nih.gov/pmc/articles/PMC4360007/

5   Jun, Y.S., Kang, P., Min, S.S., Lee, J.M., Kim, H.K., Seol, G.H. (2013). Effect of eucalyptus oil inhalation on pain and inflammatory responses after total knee replacement: a randomized clinical trial. *Evid Based Complement Alternat Med.* Retrieved from http://www.ncbi.nlm.nih.gov/pubmed/23853660

6   Sudhoff, H., Klenke, C., Greiner, J.F.W., Müller, J., Brotzmann, V., Ebmeyer, J., Kaltschmidt, B., Kaltschmidt, C. (2015). 1,8-Cineol Reduces Mucus-Production in a Novel Human Ex Vivo Model of Late Rhinosinusitis. *PLoS One.* Retrieved from http://www.ncbi.nlm.nih.gov/pmc/articles/PMC4514714/

7   Suhail, M.M., Wu, W., Cao, A., Mondalek, F.G., Fung, K.M., Shih, P.T., Fang, Y.T., Woolley, C., Young, G., Lin, H.K. (2011, December). Boswellia sacra essential oil induces tumor cell-specific apoptosis and suppresses tumor aggressiveness in cultured human breast cancer cells. *BMC Complement Altern Med.* Retrieved from http://www.ncbi.nlm.nih.gov/pubmed/22171782

8   Khosravi Samani, M., Mahmoodian, H., Moghadamnia, A., Poorsattar Bejeh Mir, A., Chitsazan, M. (2011). The effect of Frankincense in the treatment of moderate plaque-induced

gingivitis: a double blinded randomized clinical trial. *Daru*. Retrieved from http://www.ncbi.nlm.nih.gov/pubmed/22615671

9   Sebai, H., Selmi, S., Rtibi, K., Souli, A., Gharbi, N., Sakly, M. (2013, December 28). Lavender (Lavandula stoechas L.) essential oils attenuate hyperglycemia and protect against oxidative stress in alloxan-induced diabetic rats. *Lipids Health Dis*. Retrieved from http://www.ncbi.nlm.nih.gov/pmc/articles/PMC3880178/

10 Hossein Koulivand, P., Khaleghi Ghadiri, M., Gorji, A. (2013). Lavender and the Nervous System. *Evid Based Complement Alternat Med*. Retrieved from http://www.ncbi.nlm.nih.gov/pmc/articles/PMC3612440/

11 Uehleke, B., Schaper, S., Dienel, A., Schlaefke, S., Stange, R. (2012, June 15). Phase II trial on the effects of Silexan in patients with neurasthenia, post-traumatic stress disorder or somatization disorder. Unbound MEDLINE. Retrieved from http://www.unboundmedicine.com/medline/citation/22475718/Phase_II _trial_on_the_effects_of_Silexan_in_patients_with_neurasthenia _post_traumatic_stress_disorder_or_somatization_disorder_

12 Yavari Kia, P., Safajou, F., Shahnazi, M., Nazemiyeh, H. (2014, March). The effect of lemon inhalation aromatherapy on nausea and vomiting of pregnancy: a double-blinded, randomized, controlled clinical trial. *Iran Red Crescent Med J*. Retrieved from http://www.ncbi.nlm.nih.gov/pubmed/24829772

13 Komiya, M., Takeuchi, T., Harada, E. (2006, September). Lemon oil vapor causes an anti-stress effect via modulating the 5-HT and DA activities in mice. *Behav Brain Res*. Retrieved from http://www.ncbi.nlm.nih.gov/pubmed/16780969

14 Enshaieh, S., Jooya, A., Siadat, A.H., Iraji, F. (2007, January). The efficacy of 5% topical tea tree oil gel in mild to moderate acne vulgaris: a randomized, double-blind placebo-controlled study. *Indian J Dermatol Venereol Leprol*. Retrieved from http://www.ncbi.nlm.nih.gov/pubmed/17314442

15 Ramage, G., Milligan, S., Lappin, D.F., Sherry, L., Sweeney, P., Williams, C., Bagg, J., Culshaw, S. (2012, June 18). Antifungal, Cytotoxic, and Immunomodulatory Properties of Tea Tree Oil and Its Derivative Components: Potential Role in Management of Oral Candidosis in Cancer Patients. *Front Microbiol*. Retrieved from http://www.ncbi.nlm.nih.gov/pmc/articles/PMC3376416/

16 Chen, Y., Zhou, C., Ge, Z., Liu, Y., Liu, Y., Fend, W., Wei, T. 2013. Composition and potential anticancer activities of essential oils obtained from myrrh and frankincense. *Oncology Letters*, 6(4), 1140–1146. Retrieved from http://doi.org/10.3892/ol.2013.1520

17   Haffor, A.S. (2010, March). Effect of myrrh (Commiphora molmol) on leukocyte levels before and during healing from gastric ulcer or skin injury. *J Immunotoxicol*. Retrieved from http://www.ncbi .nlm.nih.gov/pubmed/19995243

18   Qiu, P., Dong, P., Guan, H., Li, S., Ho, C.-T., Pan, M.-H., McClements, D. J. and Xiao, H. (2010). Inhibitory effects of 5-hydroxy polymethoxyflavones on colon cancer cells. *Mol. Nutr. Food Res.*, 54: S244–S252. doi: 10.1002/mnfr.200900605

19   Igarashi, M., Ikei, H., Song, C., Miyazaki, Y. (2014, December). Effects of olfactory stimulation with rose and orange oil on prefrontal cortex activity. *Complement Ther Med*. Retrieved from http://www .ncbi.nlm.nih.gov/pubmed/25453523

20   Sienkiewicz, M., Wasiela, M., Głowacka, A. (2012). The antibacterial activity of oregano essential oil (Origanum heracleoticum L.) against clinical strains of Escherichia coli and Pseudomonas aeruginosa. *Med Dosw Mikrobiol*. Retrieved from http://www.ncbi .nlm.nih.gov/pubmed/23484421

21   Gilling, D.H., Kitajima, M., Torrey, J.R., Bright. K.R. (2014, May). Antiviral efficacy and mechanisms of action of oregano essential oil and its primary component carvacrol against murine norovirus. *J Appl Microbiol*. Retrieved from http://www.ncbi.nlm .nih.gov/pubmed/24779581

22   Cappello, G., Spezzaferro, M., Grossi, L., Manzoli, L., Marzio, L. (2007, June). Peppermint oil (Mintoil) in the treatment of irritable bowel syndrome: a prospective double blind placebo-controlled randomized trial. *Dig Liver Dis*. Retrieved from http://www.ncbi .nlm.nih.gov/pubmed/17420159

23   Göbel, H., Schmidt, G., Soyka, D. (1994, June). Effect of peppermint and eucalyptus oil preparations on neurophysiological and experimental algesimetric headache parameters. *Cephalalgia*. Retrieved from http://www.ncbi.nlm.nih.gov/pubmed/7954745

24   Moss, M., Oliver, L. (2012). Plasma 1,8-cineole correlates with cognitive performance following exposure to rosemary essential oil aroma. *Therapeutic Advances in Psychopharmacology*, 2(3), 103–113. http://doi.org/10.1177/2045125312436573

25   Luqman, S., Dwivedi, G.R., Darokar, M.P., Kalra. A., Khanuja, S.P. (2007, September). Potential of rosemary oil to be used in drug-resistant infections. *Altern Ther Health Med*. Retrieved from http: //www.ncbi.nlm.nih.gov/pubmed/17900043

26   Takemoto, H., Ito, M., Shiraki, T., Yagura, T., Honda, G. (2008, January). Sedative effects of vapor inhalation of agarwood oil and spikenard extract and identification of their active components.

J Nat Med. Retrieved from http://www.ncbi.nlm.nih.gov/pubmed/18404340

27 Gottumukkala, V.R., Annamalai, T., Mukhopadhyay, T. (2011). Phytochemical investigation and hair growth studies on the rhizomes of Nardostachys jatamansi DC. *Pharmacognosy Magazine,* 7(26), 146–150. Retrieved from http://doi .org/10.4103/0973-1296.80674

28 Braden, R., Reichow, S., Halm, MA. (2009, December 24). The use of the essential oil lavandin to reduce preoperative anxiety in surgical patients. *Journal of PeriAnesthesia Nursing.* Retrieved from http://www.ncbi.nlm.nih.gov/pubmed/19962101

29 Tournaire, M., Theau-Yonneau, A. (2007, December 4). Complementary and Alternative Approaches to Pain Relief During Labor. *Evid Based Complement Alternat Med.* Retrieved from http://www.ncbi.nlm.nih.gov/pmc/articles/PMC2176140/

30 Glaser, G. (2002, December 17). Doctors Rethinking Treatments for Sick Sinuses. Wayne State University. Retrieved from http://www .nytimes.com/2002/12/17/health/doctors-rethinking-treatments-for-sick-sinuses.html?pagewanted=all

31 Cingi, C., Conk-Dalay, M., Cakli, H., Bal, C. (2008, October). The effects of spirulina on allergic rhinitis. *Eur Arch Otorhinolaryngol.* Retrieved from http://www.ncbi.nlm.nih.gov/pubmed/18343939

32 Kasper, S. (2013, November). An orally administered lavandula oil preparation (Silexan) for anxiety disorder and related conditions: an evidence based review. *Int J Psychiatry Clin Pract.* Retrieved from http://www.ncbi. nlm.nih.gov/pubmed/?term=International+Journal+of+ Psychiatry+in+Clinical+Practice+lavender+anxiety

33 Cooley, K., Szczurko, O., Perri, D., Mills, E., Bernhardt, B., Zhou, Q., Seely, D. (2009, August 31). Naturopathic Care for Anxiety: A Randomized Controlled Trial ISRCTN78958974. *PLoS One.* Retrieved from http://www.ncbi.nlm.nih.gov/pmc/articles /PMC2729375/

34 Thomson, M., Al-Qattan, KK., Al-Sawan, SM., Alnaqeeb, MA., Khan, I., Ali, M. (2002 December). The use of ginger (Zingiber officinale Rosc.) as a potential anti-inflammatory and antithrombotic agent. *Prostaglandins Leukot Essent Fatty Acids.* Retrieved by http://www .ncbi.nlm.nih.gov/pubmed/12468270

35 Jeena K, Liju VB, Kuttan R. (2013, March). Antioxidant, anti-inflammatory and antinociceptive activities of essential oil from ginger. *Indian J Physiol Pharmacol. Pubmed, 24020099.* Retrieved from http://www.ncbi.nlm.nih.gov/pubmed/24020099

36   Reed, GW., Leung., K., Rossetti, RG., Vanbuskirk, S., Sharp, JT., Zurier, RB. (2014, March 19). Treatment of rheumatoid arthritis with marine and botanical oils: an 18-month, randomized, and double-blind trial. *Evid Based Complement Alternat Med.* Retrieved by http://www.ncbi.nlm.nih.gov/pubmed/24803948

37   Pattanayak, P., Behera, P., Das, D., Panda, S.K. (2010, June). Ocimum sanctum Linn. A reservoir plant for therapeutic applications: An overview. *Pharmacogn Rev.* Retrieved from http://www.ncbi.nlm.nih.gov/pmc/articles/PMC3249909/

38   Misni, N., Nor, ZM., Ahmad, R. (2016, June). New Candidates for Plant-Based Repellents Against Aedes aegypti. *J Am Mosq Control Assoc.* Retrieved from http://www.ncbi.nlm.nih.gov/pubmed/27280349

39   (2016). Upper Respiratory Infection (URI or Common Cold). *Hopkins Medicine.* Retrieved from http://www.hopkinsmedicine.org/healthlibrary/conditions/pediatrics/upper_respiratory_infection_uri_or_common_cold_90,P02966/

40   Gill, TA., Li, J., Saenger, M., Scofield, SR. (2016, June 2). Thymol-based submicron emulsions exhibit antifungal activity against Fusarium graminearum and inhibit Fusarium head blight in wheat. *J Appl Microbiol.* Retrieved from http://www.ncbi.nlm.nih.gov/pubmed/27253757

41   Hamada, M., Uezu, K., Matsushita, J., Yamamoto, S., Kishino, Y. (2002, April). Distribution and immune responses resulting from oral administration of D-limonene in rats. *J Nutr Sci Vitaminol (Tokyo).* Retrieved from http://www.ncbi.nlm.nih.gov/pubmed/12171437

42   Lissiman, E., Bhasale, AL., Cohen, M. (2014, November 11). Garlic for the common cold. *Cochrane Database Syst Rev.* Retrieved from http://www.ncbi.nlm.nih.gov/pubmed/25386977

43   Hongratanaworakit, T. (2011, August). Aroma-therapeutic effects of massage blended essential oils on humans. *Nat Prod Commun.* Retrieved from http://www.ncbi.nlm.nih.gov/pubmed/21922934

44   Conrad, P., Adams, C. (2012, August). The effects of clinical aromatherapy for anxiety and depression in the high risk postpartum woman - a pilot study. *Complement Ther Clin Pract.* Retrieved from http://www.ncbi.nlm.nih.gov/pubmed/22789792

45   Göbel, H., Fresenius, J., Heinze, A., Dworschak, M., Soyka, D. (1996, August). Effectiveness of Oleum menthae piperitae and paracetamol in therapy of headache of the tension type. *Nervenarzt.* Retrieved from http://www.ncbi.nlm.nih.gov/pubmed/8805113

46 Sasannejad, P., Saeedi, M., Shoeibi, A., Gorji, A., Abbasi, M., Foroughipour, M. (2012). Lavender essential oil in the treatment of migraine headache: a placebo-controlled clinical trial. *Eur Neurol.* Retrieved from http://www.ncbi.nlm.nih.gov/pubmed/22517298

47 Assarzadegan, F., Asgarzadeh, S., Hatamabadi, HR., Shahrami, A., Tabatabaey, A., Asgarzadeh, M. (2016, September). Serum concentration of magnesium as an independent risk factor in migraine attacks: a matched case-control study and review of the literature. *Int Clin Psychopharmacol.* Retrieved from http://www.ncbi.nlm.nih.gov/pubmed/27140442

48 Ernst, E., Pittler, MH. (2000, December). The efficacy and safety of feverfew (Tanacetum parthenium L.): an update of a systematic review. *Public Health Nutr.* Retrieved from http://www.ncbi.nlm.nih.gov/pubmed/11276299

49 Ehrlich, S. (2014, July 6). Peppermint. *A.D.A.M., Inc.* Retrieved from http://umm.edu/health/medical/altmed/herb/peppermint

50 Liju, VB., Jeena, K., Kuttan, R. (2015). Gatroprotective Activity of Essential Oils from Turmeric and Ginger. J Basic Clin Physiol *Pharmacol.* Retrieved from http://www.ncbi.nlm.nih.gov/pubmed/24756059

51 Jaber, R. (2002, June). Respiratory and allergic diseases: from upper respiratory tract infections to asthma. *Prim Care.* Retrieved from http://www.ncbi.nlm.nih.gov/pubmed/?term=frankincense+essential+oil+blood+cell

52 Faramarzi, S., Bozorgmehrirard, M.H., Khaki, A., Moomivand, H., Saeid Ezati, M., Rasoulinezhad, S., Bahnamiri, A.J., Dizaji, B.R. (2013). *Annals of Biological Research.* Retrieved from http://scholarsresearchlibrary.com/ABR-vol4-iss6/ABR-2013-4-6-290-294.pdf

53 Béjaoui, A., Chaabane, H., Jemli, M., Boulila, A., Boussaid, M. (2013, December 1). Essential Oil Composition and Antibacterial Activity of Origanum vulgare subsp. glandulosum Desf. at Different Phenological Stages. *J Med Food.* Retrieved from http://www.ncbi.nlm.nih.gov/pmc/articles/PMC3868303/

54 Bento, A.F., Marcon, R., Dutra, R.C., Claudino, R.F., Cola, M., Pereira Leite, D.F., Calixto, J.B. (2011, March). ß-Caryophyllene Inhibits Dextran Sulfate Sodium-Induced Colitis in Mice through CB2 Receptor Activation and PPARγ Pathway. *Am J Pathol.* Retrieved from http://www.ncbi.nlm.nih.gov/pmc/articles/PMC3070571/

55 Chaudhari, L.K., Jawale, B.A., Sharma, S., Sharma, H., Kumar, C.D., Kulkarni, P.A. (2012, January 1). Antimicrobial activity of commercially available essential oils against Streptococcus

mutans. *J Contemp Dent Pract.* Retrieved from http://www.ncbi
.nlm.nih.gov/pubmed/22430697

56 Miller, S.C. (2005, September). Echinacea: a Miracle Herb
against Aging and Cancer? Evidence In vivo in Mice. *Evid Based
Complement Alternat Med.* Retrieved from http://www.ncbi.nlm
.nih.gov/pmc/articles/PMC1193558/

57 Sosaa, S., Altiniera, G., Politib, M., Bracab, A., Morellib, I., Della
Loggiaa, R. (2004, February 2). Extracts and constituents of
Lavandula multifida with topical anti-inflammatory activity.
Phytomedicine. Retrieved from http://www.sciencedirect.com
/science/article/pii/S0944711304001412

58 Chandola, HC., Chakraborty, A. (2009, October). Fibromyalgia
and myofascial pain syndrome-a dilemma. *Indian J Anaesth.*
Retrieved from http://www.ncbi.nlm.nih.gov/pmc/articles/
PMC2900090/#CIT21

59 Pillai, A.K., Sharma, K.K., Gupta, Y.K., Bakhshi, S. (2011, February).
Anti-emetic effect of ginger powder versus placebo as an add-on
therapy in children and young adults receiving high emetogenic
chemotherapy. *Pediatr Blood Cancer.* Retrieved from http://www.
ncbi.nlm.nih.gov/pubmed/20842754

60 Prakash, P., Gupta, N. (2005, April). Therapeutic uses of
Ocimum sanctum Linn (Tulsi) with a note on eugenol and its
pharmacological actions: a short review. *Indian J Physiol Pharmacol.*
Retrieved from http://www.ncbi.nlm.nih.gov/pubmed/16170979

61 Tayarani-Najaran, Z., Talasaz-Firoozi, E., Nasiri, R., Jalali, N.,
Hassanzadeh, M.K. (2013). Antiemetic activity of volatile oil from
Mentha spicata and Mentha × piperita in chemotherapy-induced
nausea and vomiting. *ecancer.* Retrieved from http://ecancer.org/
journal/7/290-antiemetic-activity-of-volatile-oil-from-mentha-
spicata-and-mentha-piperita-in-chemotherapy-induced-nausea-
and-vomiting.php

62 Ogden, C.L., Carroll, M.D., Kit, B.K., Flegal, K.M. (2012). How many
people are affected by/at risk for obesity and overweight? *Centers
for Disease Control and Prevention.* Retrieved from https://www.
nichd.nih.gov/health/topics/obesity/conditioninfo/Pages/risk.aspx

63 (2011). Health Benefits of Black Pepper Essential Oil. *Organic Facts.*
Retrieved from https://www.organicfacts.net/health-benefits/
essential-oils/health-benefits-of-black-pepper-essential-oil.html

64 Shen, J., Niijima, A., Tanida, M., Horii, Y., Maeda, K., Nagai, K. (2005,
June 3). Olfactory stimulation with scent of grapefruit oil affects
autonomic nerves, lipolysis and appetite in rats. *Neurosci Lett.*
Retrieved from http://www.ncbi.nlm.nih.gov/pubmed/15862904

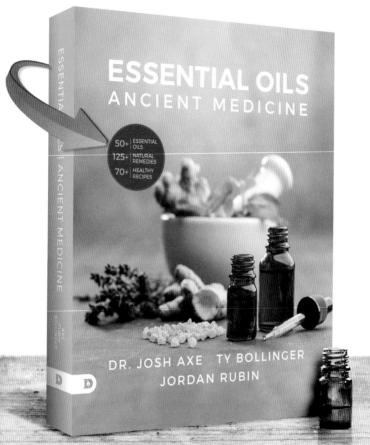